Raw Paleo

Raw Paleo

The Extreme Advantages of Eating Paleo Foods in the Raw

Includes Health Wisdom and Recipes

MELISSA HENIG & ALFREDO URSO, PhD

ISBN: 0692623779
ISBN 13: 9780692623770

Warning / Disclaimer

On the *Raw Paleo* way of eating it's important to only eat ORGANIC animal foods that are GRASS-FED or PASTURE-RAISED.

Testimonials

Melissa is highly creative in how she designs her unique raw paleo recipes. She takes raw butter, which is a super healthy fat, and creates delicious mouthwatering desserts that actually heal your body. She makes eating raw fat a tasty and fun experience.

    - Marilyn Brown, B.S.

For 15 years I diligently worked on stabilizing hypoglycemia and anemia. Then, unexpectedly, within 48 hours of enjoying raw paleo foods these symptoms disappeared. I also felt satiated for the first time in my life, and noticed that I did not crave sweets anymore. My cravings for processed foods also decreased. My body is now in the best shape ever. I no longer need to take digestive enzymes or many supplements. This is the best feel-good food ever!

    - Sarah Flowers

When I was 20 years old I developed headaches and learned to live with them until I was 30. The headaches later turned into regular migraines. I would have to miss days out of my life because I could not function with the migraines. Fed up with taking medications, I started drinking raw milk and also improved the way I ate. I soon noticed a reduction in the migraines, and after two years they became rare. I learned that my body was deprived of healthy raw fat. Raw milk saved my life and helped me achieve a lifestyle that I love.

- Kippy Miller

Ever since I've started eating raw meat I've had more energy, and now look forward to each meal.

- Caroline Younger

I've been eating raw meat for 25 years, and as a result have healed several symptoms and improved my health. I can tell you that bacteria are your friends. Without bacteria your body could not function.

- Louis Canjemi

I've eaten about a dozen quality raw eggs every day for a year and a half. Since then my health has improved and I haven't experienced any sick days. Cholesterol, our bodies need it and cannot survive without it.

- Danny Scholla

I have phenomenal energy, mental clarity, and sleep better at night after starting to eat raw meat.

- Max Kane

I usually eat 3 whole raw eggs in the morning because they digest easily and quickly in their raw form, which allows me workout soon after I wake up. I've tried other foods but can never keep them down. Only raw eggs can do the trick.

- Mary Smith

I've just had a beautiful baby boy and ate raw paleo while pregnant. I enjoyed eating raw bison, raw bison liver, raw beef, raw fish, roe, raw cheese, raw eggs, raw milk, raw kefir, raw yogurt, raw coconut cream, fresh green juice, and lots of raw butter. I had a complication-free natural birth, with no meds. I was in labor for 4 hours, and had the baby an hour after arriving at the birth center. I believe all these amazing lubricating fats helped keep me calm, happy, and focused.

   - Nicole Lienemann

Dedication

I dedicate this book to my wonderful Mother who started me on my health journey at the tender age of thirteen, and who still supports and inspires me daily. I thank you for all your encouragement.

I give special thanks to Dr. Alfredo Urso for generously giving your time in writing this book. Your wisdom of wellness and of life, together with your Intuition, has been a blessing to me. It was great working with you through the editing process, and I will continue to carry this wisdom with me on my life's journey.

The late Aajonus Vonderplanitz changed the way I look at food. He was a true pioneer in the area of raw omnivorous food. His dedicated work has healed numerous diseases and changed countless lives. Thank you for paving the way with all your passion and hard work.

Kippy Miller's instinctive nature, kindness, and generosity have been a gift to me. I've learned many tips and tricks from you. Thank you kindly.

Max Wolf's dedication to the raw lifestyle is truly inspiring. I'm in awe of your raw recipes and kitchen skills. Much gratitude.

Ruthie Paniagua, I thank you for your unconditional love and support.

Anthony Farano, my dear friend, who is a genius in the kitchen and can meet a need before it's seen. I've learned many recipes and skills from your God-given culinary gifts. I'm grateful to you.

Contents

The Extreme Advantages
of Eating Paleo Foods Raw

Raw omnivorous foods, unlike cooked omnivorous foods, have all of their inherent nutritional, chemical, enzymatic, probiotic, energetic, and DNA structures intact. Since these foods are still in their original nature-made state your body can easily utilize all of these healthful components found in the food.

Nature intends that we eat foods in the same form that she makes them. She is wiser than the entire scientific community combined!

Unlike cooked foods, raw paleo foods contain a large spectrum of probiotic species required to restore your gut microbiome. Outstanding health awaits you.

Raw paleo foods have a reputation for making you look fabulous and feel energized. Enjoy.

Enjoying the Occasional Cooked Meal

I like to eat cooked foods occasionally when eating the raw paleo way. Here are two cooking methods that allow you the pleasure of eating cooked foods periodically, without producing any of the typical toxins that form during the cooking process.

BOILING POINT METHOD

The many inherent qualities of food start to degrade and alter when cooking temperature reaches boiling point (212 degrees Fahrenheit or 100 degrees Celsius). If your body is well attuned you'll be able to taste and feel the difference of cooking below this cut off point.

SOUS VIDE METHOD

This French way of cooking literally means "under vacuum," and allows you to cook food slowly at low temperatures. Place the food into a glass mason jar, seal, and put the jar into temperature-controlled warm water. The process takes approximately 96 hours at a temperature of 140 Fahrenheit. Vegetables require a slightly higher temperature.

Preface

If you're like most people, you may be feeling unhappy with your current level of health. I understand, because I also used to feel this way. I took many vitamin pills for twenty years, but to no avail. In fact, in the long term they had adverse effects. I later learned that laboratory-made substances are foreign to the body and therefore can increase one's toxic load. Fortunately, several years later I found the answer in nature's healing foods.

I've eaten the raw paleo way for 17 years now, and feel blessed to have found such a delicious and healthful way to eat. I was surprised to see my health improve with such little effort other than enjoying my food! Even more surprising were the unexpected psychological improvements I saw in my clients who ate raw paleo.

When I first began to eat in this way I came across many cultural myths, but as I explored them one by one I realized they were untrue. Cultural myths infiltrate all areas of life, and it's up to us to investigate and distinguish fact from fiction. I came to realize that people have eaten the raw paleo way for millennia, and it makes sense that our body still needs this kind of food.

I also learned that cooked foods have **less healing potential** and **more disease potential** than their whole raw counterparts.

There are numerous health benefits to eating raw paleo foods, but one of my favorites is that these foods awaken the senses and give the body a detox edge. For example, my olfactory senses have become so keen that I can now detect the slightest amount of toxins in the air. However, sometimes these ambient toxins can't be avoided. In these instances, the following morning I always cough up some mucus. The mucus in my respiratory tract adsorbed the toxins from the prior day. Our bodies are truly smart when nourished correctly.

Raw paleo foods have awakened my body's innate survival mechanism, which helps to keep the toxic load on my body at a minimum. An entire book could be written on the countless health benefits of raw paleo foods. God has provided us with foods that, when eaten in their naturally-occurring form, give us the possibility to regain our health. This is our birthright!

In this book you'll learn how to improve your health while eating delicious raw paleo recipes designed by the queen of raw, Melissa Henig.

Many Blessings to You,

Alfredo Urso, PhD
www.LightWellness.net
Venice Beach, CA

Foreword

Melissa Henig is a master chef in my world. Her raw paleo recipes have no equal. Melissa loves raw fat, and yet has a beautiful lean body. She knows that raw fat does not make you fat but instead cleanses, heals, soothes the nerves, and all cells in the body. Melissa's favorite fat is raw butter, which is known to lubricate joints, soften the skin, and give you silky looking hair.

Melissa is highly creative in how she designs her recipes. For example, she takes raw bone marrow, which is another amazing fat, and somehow creates delicious mouthwatering desserts that heal the body. She makes eating raw fat, fun and tasty.

It's important to eat foods that are grown organically, and to avoid GMO foods at all cost. Our bodies have evolved by eating uncooked, un-heated, fresh raw food. Cooked grains became popular because they were inexpensive, and were able to get people through long isolated winters. However, grains have gotten out of hand in the modern world. They fill the belly with volume, but do not fulfill nutritional requirements.

In this wonderful book Melissa provides us with many raw paleo meat recipes. Many cultures include at least one raw meat dish in their cuisine. In the USA many people used to be comfortable eating rare or raw meat until they were told the nonsense to cook their meat until it's well done. In Texas it was almost a crime to do more than wave your steak over the barbecue.

The reason why conventionally grown meat has to be thoroughly cooked nowadays is due to the microbial contamination from filthy, unhygienic farming practices. However, nowadays farms which raise animals in a healthy and clean manner are springing up everywhere. Meat from these farmers is safe to eat whether it's rare or raw, just like in the old days.

I trust you will enjoy this book as much as I have. Eat healthy and delicious foods. Melissa can show you how!

Marilyn Brown, BS, Biological Sciences.
Certificated California Science Teacher.

An Important Note to the Reader

I consider myself a raw paleo omnivore, eating all categories of raw foods such as raw meat, raw dairy, raw eggs, raw fermented vegetables, raw seeds and nuts, raw honey, raw fresh green juice, seasonal fruits, and vegetables.

As wonderful as the current version of the paleo diet may be, the reality is that we are living in a much different world than the Paleolithic one of centuries ago. Therefore, I believe the current version of the paleo diet may have some limitations in today's world. For example, the paleo diet allows cooked and processed foods to be eaten. However, these foods do not have their original nutritional, chemical, enzymatic, probiotic, energetic, and DNA structures intact the way nature intended. This means that most of the processed and heat-altered nutrients have become less metabolically active. (1) This translates to having less available nutrition for utilization into human tissue.

We also need to make nutritional adjustments for changes that occur in the modern world, such as decreased nutrients and increased toxins in our food, water, and air. The stress from modern living further depletes our body's nutrients at an accelerated rate. Additionally, our microwaved world (EMF's) depletes our body's nutrients even further. This means that our modern bodies have a much more difficult time staying healthy than they did in the Paleolithic era. To better deal with this unnatural situation of too little nutrients and excessive toxins I include raw dairy and fresh vegetable juices.

Raw dairy supplies the body with macronutrients and micronutrients that are otherwise difficult to come by in adequate amounts. For example, the raw saturated fats protect our cells from toxins while also nourishing our tissues. Raw dairy also contains high amounts of fat-soluble vitamins that are also deficient in modern-day people. These nutrients are vitamin A, D, E, and K2. All of these nutrients are super essential for brain and nervous system function, healthy skin, strong bones, hormonal balance, and immunity. Raw dairy also contains large amounts of highly bioavailable calcium which is necessary to prevent osteoporosis, dental cavities, cramps, nerve problems, anxiety, and arthritis. Some people take these nutrients in supplement form however supplements are neither paleo, raw, or healthful. (2) Anything artificial and foreign is toxic to the body, and hence the low bioavailability of all pills.

I wrote this book for the paleo foodies, primal dieters, raw vegans, and anyone who wants to take their health to the next level. <u>This book is not about eating a 100% raw diet, but rather increasing your intake of living raw foods to a level that suits your individual makeup.</u> For some people this may be as simple as adding whole raw eggs to your daily smoothies. For optimal health I recommend eating 60 - 80% of your foods in the raw form.

Raw Paleo is the culmination of 15 years of my quest for optimal health. I'm a living testimony to the fact that the raw paleo way of eating works for me, however, a variation of this program may be more suitable for you. It's always advisable to keep an open mind, and let personal experience show you what works best for you.

Eat only ORGANIC and GRASS-FED / PASTURE-RAISED animal products.

I recommend you only eat foods that are healthy for you and the planet. All foods must be organic, grass-fed in the case of cows, and pasture-raised for chickens.

The typical large scale factory farms are toxic for animals, people, and the planet. By supporting healthy and happy farms we decrease the demand for the inhumane, filthy, and stinky factory farms. I drive past these farms on some freeways, and the stench of death lingers for miles.

I believe that we're all part of the circle of life; that life isn't possible without death. I cherish and am grateful for the sacred gift that animals give us with their flesh. I nourish myself with the exact amount of raw meat my body needs, and no more.

Wherever you are on your health journey, from the bottom of my heart, I wish you everlasting health.

Your healthy friend,
Melissa Henig

The Food

A few years ago my mother and I were having lunch in sunny Venice, California. Later that afternoon I received a call from her saying how beautiful I looked. She had noticed that my cheekbones had become more prominent thereby making me look younger and more vital. I replied, "Thank you, the credit goes to my raw paleo diet."

For several years I've provided my raw omnivorous foods for sale at local farmers markets. My customers have commented on my glowing skin and the muscle tone of my arms. Some even ask if I've lost weight. "What's your secret?" they ask. I simply tell them I've been eating raw paleo foods such as grass-fed raw butter, grass-fed raw meat, and drinking a lot of green juice. You wouldn't believe the looks I get when I tell them that I eat one pound of raw butter per week. I love the shock value.... and the butter. In fact, raw butter was the enjoyable "bridge" that helped me to go from raw vegan to raw paleo.

One

MY JOURNEY FROM RAW VEGAN TO RAW PALEO

(I) *Raw Vegan Diet*

I grew up in a health-conscious home where I drank carrot juice and ate plenty of salads. A radical shift came in 2009 while living in Chicago. I remember seeing an advertisement posted at my local health food store for a raw food class. It sparked my interest and I quickly signed up. I was so inspired by the glow of the women who were teaching the class that I dove head first into the raw vegan diet. The next morning I ordered a Vitamix blender, food processor, and a dehydrator. I was excited to learn about this new raw diet, and started making all kinds of raw vegan recipes.

My new raw vegan diet meant that I eliminated all hydrogenated oils, factory farmed foods, non-organic foods, grains, legumes, refined sugars, and all processed foods. I remember feeling so energetic and healthy from eating fresh live foods. Life seemed great with my newfound energy.

About one year later, and to my surprise, I started to lose most of my newfound energy. What a disappointment! Some time afterwards,

I started noticing symptoms which I learned were to due to nutrient deficiencies. My nails became brittle and sometimes even chipped off. I experienced some muscle loss, gas, anxiety, and toothaches. I always felt hungry and cold. I felt like a balloon; voluminously full but nutritionally empty. Raw vegan got me on the right path, but I knew that something was missing.

I remember binging on large amounts of dates while trying to satiate an insatiable hunger. Unfortunately, to no avail, the hunger would not go away. My teeth started developing problems from all the date sugar. I also began having mood swings from the excessive amounts of date sugar. I decided to ditch the dates and instead started eating raw nuts. Unfortunately, the raw nuts were difficult to digest. I later learned that nuts contain high levels of phytic acid which is an anti-nutrient. They also contain high amounts of omega 6 fats, which when eaten in access cause inflammation in the body.

Something needed to change, and very quickly. My answer came in the form of Rawesome, a local raw omnivore food store in Venice, California. I was still eating a raw vegan diet, but was shopping at Rawesome for my veggies, fruit, raw oils, and some coconut water kefir. I somehow knew that I was losing out on so many delicious goodies in this unique shop. Oh… was I missing out on the land of milk and honey.

I shopped at Rawesome twice weekly and started speaking with fellow shoppers about health. Rawesome had a table with non-vegan samples, such as raw cheese, which I one day timidly tasted. Several weeks later the local folks introduced me to the raw primal diet, which included raw meat and raw dairy. Having lived as a raw vegan for one year I could relate to the raw aspect, but raw meat seemed like a stretch for me. Eager to improve my vitality I remained intrigued and open-minded. I now know that life is fulfilling and delicious when I'm open-minded. Yum! I now eat raw banana cream butter pie.

While continuing to explore these delicious new raw foods at Rawesome I learned that the critically essential omega 3 fats and fat-soluble vitamins A, D, and K2 were missing from my current raw vegan diet. These important fat-soluble vitamins are not found in plants. Sure, I was getting vitamin K1 in green leafy vegetables, but I was missing out on the valuable vitamin K2 which is primarily found in raw animal fats such as eggs, butter, and cheese. Vitamin K2 has the ability to direct calcium to where it's needed in the body, for example the bones and teeth. Vitamin K2 also plays an important role in proper facial development in children, and removes plaque from the arteries. I also learned that my vegan foods were deficient in raw cholesterol and other important nutrients, such as iron and vitamin B12. I feel blessed to be eating these important nutrients nowadays.

One of the most important things I learned is that our brain and nervous system require <u>raw</u> animal fat in order to function optimally. This means eating plenty of raw eggs, raw butter, raw cream, and raw animal meats. Unfortunately, raw vegan fats cannot effectively nourish the brain and nervous system due to their lack of fat-soluble vitamins. Raw vegan fats such as avocados, coconuts, and olives are great at nourishing other areas of the body. On the raw vegan diet I was starving my brain and nervous system of these healthy raw animal fats. This could explain the anxiety and ungrounded feeling that I was experiencing on the raw vegan diet.

Within two weeks of including raw dairy in my diet, I noticed wonderful changes in my body. I felt nourished, satiated, strong, and happy. My nutrient deficiencies after one year of raw veganism were so severe that when I first ate raw butter I couldn't seem to get enough of it. It tasted and felt so good to my body. I noticed that my constant craving for food started to diminish, my nails got stronger, bruises disappeared, thinking became clearer, and I slept much better. My diet nowadays is so nutrient-dense and satisfying that I periodically have to remind myself to eat. I like how a couple of pieces of raw cheese easily satisfy my hunger. What a relief not to have to force mounds of kale into my body, and still feel hungry.

Raw butter has made my skin soft and lubricated my joints. Dry skin and stiff joints are common symptoms amongst my vegan friends. The raw milk has been great at strengthening my bones and teeth. The raw meat has added muscle to my entire body, making me look young and toned. I love how sexy and feminine I feel.

(II) *Raw Primal Diet*

My second introduction to raw diets was the Primal Diet by Aajonus Vonderplanitz, a pioneer of the raw omnivorous diet. (3) Aajonus was a nutritional pioneer many years ahead of his peers. On this diet people eat a large variety of omnivorous raw foods. Many people come to the raw primal diet after trying numerous eating programs, drugs, supplements, and other modalities that have not worked. Mr. Vonderplanitz successfully healed himself of ADD, autism, blood cancer, and bone cancer. He has helped hundreds of people to heal from "terminal" conditions which are documented in his book titled *We Want to Live*.

(III) *Traditional Diets*

I also found myself drawn to the work of Dr. Weston A. Price. He was a successful dentist in the 1930's who studied the eating patterns and resulting health of numerous traditional cultures across the globe. He found direct correlations between foods eaten and the health of the entire body, including teeth and dental arches. Every native diet contained animal products, and had no refined or denatured foods.

Dr. Price noticed that cultures eating whole foods were healthy, strong, and attractive. They were free from the numerous modern-day diseases, dental decay, and mental illnesses. People were able to easily conceive and painless childbirth was the norm. Nowadays, when parents follow a Weston A. Price diet for a substantial number of years their children have naturally straight teeth and broad faces. When modern-day parents eat modern processed foods their kids experience facial bone loss and often-times need braces.

In his book *Nutrition and Physical Degeneration*, Dr. Price reports that traditional people mainly ate animal fat, animal protein, organ meats, raw dairy, and fermented vegetables. (4) He concluded that the diets of non-industrialized cultures contained at least 4 times the amount of miner-als found in the Standard American Diet. Their diets also contained 10 times the amount of water-soluble vitamins and fat-soluble vitamins. Fat-soluble vitamins (A, D, and K2) are exclusive to animal fats.

Dr. Price observed that after eating processed, nutrient-depleted foods these cultures started to develop systemic skeletal deformities. These were narrow hips, small shoulders, slender face, loss of cheek-bones, receding chin, constricted nostrils, small jaw, and narrow dental arches with overcrowded teeth. These modern maladies are not natural, and only came about after the introduction of denatured foods.

Dr. Price additionally found that chronic undernourishment also re-sulted in ailments such as reproductive disorders, obesity, diabetes, and heart disease. Dr. Price believed that if nutritional deficiencies were not corrected, children with minor mental instabilities later developed pathological mental disorders. He found that when cultural undernourishment spanned several generations, moral degradation also increase. Such spiritual erosion has become increasingly common in the modern world.

It's time to get back to eating the way nature intended, so ditch the "poison in pretty packages" such as low-fat, sugar-free, and no-cholesterol foods. Real whole foods are the only way to achieve good health and longevity.

(IV) Paleo Diet

After studying and experiencing the prior three diets I was drawn to the paleo diet. The Paleolithic diet is based on food that our human ancestors most likely ate such as meat, eggs, tubers, nuts, vegetables, and berries. Our ancestors controlled gene expression and health by following a natural diet and living in a clean environment. Nowadays we can do the same.

People who eat the cooked version of the paleo diet have successfully healed many modern diseases such as diabetes, chronic fatigue, bowel disorders, brain problems, inflammation, autoimmune disease, and cardiovascular disease. However, I realized that many people on this diet a lot of cooked food, which means that they are ingesting many kinds of toxins formed by the cooking process (more info see Raw Meat Chapter). Another thing that doesn't resonate with me is that some paleo folk are only interested in whether a food is paleo or not. They don't pay attention to the quality of the food; whether it's been highly denatured or not. I've seen paleo followers eating canned, packaged, and other denatured stuff.

Two

Labels Cause Nutrient Deficiencies

People can sometimes unknowingly restrict their nutrient intake by using labels that cut out entire food groups. Labels such as fruitarian, raw vegan, vegan, vegetarian, and pescatarian have become increasingly popular. "I can't eat that, I'm a pescatarian." What the heck is a pescatarian anyway? I hadn't even heard of it until I moved to California.

Research shows that humans evolved by eating a varied omnivorous diet. Therefore, if you omit any food group you could be causing a deficiency of essential nutrients. Simply put, restrictive labels restrict nutrients. There's a lot of freedom, and health, to be found when you lose the label. Freedom is wellness!

~ *Restrictive labels restrict nutrients.* ~

For me Raw Paleo is not a restrictive label because it includes the entire range of raw foods that our omnivorous ancestors ate. My diet only restricts two food groups that our ancestors did <u>not</u> eat. These foods are grains and legumes, which were first cultivated only 12,000 years ago. Have compassion for yourself if your body craves these two food groups periodically. I occasionally indulge in these foods and enjoy them.

A case in point is a close friend who had adopted the vegetarian label for 14 years, and had later developed intestinal bloating, digestive problems, anxiety, a thyroid imbalance, and also felt stressed. One day when I was making raw bison tartare for lunch she told me that she had low levels of iron and B vitamins. I took a bite of the raw meat and told her about the numerous health benefits of raw meat. For example, the highly absorbable form of vitamin B12 can help with the anxiety she was experiencing. To my surprise she eagerly took a bite, and nowadays loves eating raw meat. She regularly orders bison tartare from me and says that her body craves it and feels great after eating it. Her new label is "I'm a vegetarian except when I eat Melissa's raw bison." After only several weeks of eating raw meat many of her symptoms significantly improved.

What habits are you picking up from your friends? Remember that you become like the top five people you're around, so choose wisely. In the above example, my friend became a little more like me.

Another friend of mine had labeled herself as vegan for 9 years, and suffered with terrible migraines and tension headaches. On her plant-based diet she obviously wasn't eating any raw cholesterol or raw animal fats, which are required by the brain and nervous system. Raw cholesterol and raw animal fats are known to simultaneously cleanse and nourish the brain and nervous system. Like other vegan friends, as soon as they introduced raw animal fats into their diets the migraines disappeared.

Recently a vegan client sent me a text saying she was unable to raise her arms above her head due to shoulder pain and stiffness. She wanted to spend $200 to see a doctor. I said, "How is he going to put raw fat and nourishment into your cells?" I kept pleading with her to eat some raw fat. "Please eat just one raw egg and some raw butter," I told her. "Your body needs it really badly." "How far would your car get without oil," I asked? A few days later she picked up some raw paleo chocolate pudding that I make from raw butter, raw eggs, raw cacao powder, and raw honey. Within a few days her shoulder pain and stiffness had improved. The reason why the raw butter helped her shoulder is because it contains the *Wulzen factor,* an anti-stiffness nutrient that's only found when butter and cream are in their raw state. Raw fats are nature's lubrication material and therefore play a major role in joint health. Raw paleo chocolate pudding is a delicious way for newcomers to get raw eggs and raw butter into their body.

~ *Freedom is wellness.* ~

Living without labels gives you the freedom to eat the wide variety of foods and nutrients that your body requires. Your Instinct can guide you as to how much and how often you need to eat a particular food. This method is very accurate once you're in tune with your body. Take particular note of any signs and symptoms because they're important indicators of your nutritional status. Over time you will become increasingly more in tune with your Instinct, and know when, what, and how much to eat. You'll then find that labels are not required.

Three

Fresh Organic Raw Paleo Foods

Hippocrates, the father of modern medicine, is known to have said, "Let food be thy medicine and medicine be thy food." I agree fully, and that's why I choose to eat real food. It just makes sense to eat what disease-free people have traditionally eaten. Famous American physician, Henry Bieler, MD claimed that real food is your best medicine. (5) The diets of healthy non-industrialized people did not contain refined foods or any processed ingredients. They did not use canned foods, low-fat anything, hydrogenated vegetable oils, protein powders, synthetic vitamins, additives, colorings, and especially no GMO's.

Don't Denature Nature

I've come to realize that to denature nature is unwise. Raw paleo foods are typically eaten in their naturally occurring state which is unheated and unprocessed. They are never cooked, pasteurized, homogenized, irradiated, microwaved, chemicalized, or altered in any way. Whole raw paleo foods eaten in their naturally occurring state have a high bioavailability, which means that your body can easily absorb and utilize the nutrients.

Living Enzymes

Another great quality of raw omnivorous foods is that they still have their full quota of enzymes. Enzymes are catalysts which are important because they make all biochemical processes possible. Our body has a store of enzymes which can become depleted over time. When enzymes are depleted, every bodily function comes to a halt; diseases start to manifest. (6) Raw foods help to make the body's inherent enzymes last longer. This happens because when you are digesting your food your body uses the enzymes inherent in the food, rather than depleting its own store of enzymes.

Because of the inherent enzymes found in raw foods they are able to easily digest. This leaves people with <u>more energy</u> and less of the typical post-meal discomforts like lethargy, gas, and bloating. Enzymes are also systemic healers and can contribute to healing all kinds of diseases.

Probiotics

All raw foods, including omnivorous raw foods, are teaming with numerous beneficial microorganisms: bacteria, viruses, and fungi. When food is grown in an organic sustainable manner the resulting microorganisms are pro-life; in other words they are probiotics. These food probiotics are truly broad spectrum, unlike store bought probiotics which only contain several strains.

Without microorganisms humans cannot sustain health because microorganisms are required for all cellular processes. For example, cells in our body are continually dying and need to be replaced by new cells with the help of microorganisms. Aging is accelerated without these naturally occurring probiotics. Eating raw foods means that you will have an ample supply of these rejuvenative probiotics. The naturally occurring probiotics in raw foods are anti-aging.

~ The naturally occurring probiotics in raw paleo foods are anti-aging. ~

Probiotics in raw paleo foods are also powerful detoxifiers. A primary function of microorganisms is to consume toxic waste that's in the body, and carry it out of the body. Therefore without sufficient amounts of pro-biotics the body can become increasingly toxic over time.

The Raw Paleo Foods:
Raw butter
Raw cheese
Raw milk
Raw cream
Raw milk kefir
Raw yogurt
Raw eggs
Raw steak tartare
Raw chicken ceviche
Raw fish ceviche and sashimi
Raw glands and organs
Raw unheated honey
Raw fresh green juice

Raw fresh coconut water (straight out of a coconut)
Raw fresh coconut cream (see coconut cream recipe in Condiment Chapter)
Raw soaked seeds
Raw soaked nuts
Fresh seasonal fruit
Raw vegetables
Raw fermented vegetables
Raw fresh herbs

Eating Cooked Foods Occasionally
I strongly advocate listening to your Instinct in order to know when to eat cooked foods. I eat very well at home, but in social situations I do the best I can. Listen to your body, because it's totally fine to eat healthy cooked food periodically.

My Favorite Cooked Foods (yours may be different):
Lightly cooked homemade traditional bone broths and soups.
Lightly sautéed organic greens cooked in coconut oil, beef tallow, or lard.
Organic sweet potatoes with raw butter as a topping.
Properly fermented sour dough bread with raw butter.
Organic Non-GMO air popped popcorn with raw butter.
Organic meals in healthy restaurants (make sure to avoid Canola, Cottonseed, and Palm oils).

Note: Since raw paleo foods are nutrient-dense and therefore cleansing, when you first begin eating them you may experience mild detox symptoms. Detoxification symptoms include: headaches, diarrhea, fatigue, nausea, muscle stiffness, joint pain, skin eruptions, and general aches and pains.

In order to avoid any uncomfortable detoxification symptoms I recommend you <u>introduce these foods gradually, one at a time</u>. **If a detox reaction still occurs simply omit all raw foods, and introduce them again after the detox is over.** Mild detox symptoms are fine and will be worth the radiant beauty and strength that follow.

Four

Fresh Organic Raw Animal Fats

Fats, in their naturally occurring raw state, are essential for the body but when denatured (heated, pasteurized, homogenized, or processed) can cause health problems. All people, as well as animals, need raw fats in order to thrive.

Raw fats are possibly the most important of the three macronutrients: fats, proteins, and carbohydrates. Furthermore, raw fats from animal sources may be the best type of raw fat. The animal type of raw fat is essential because each cell of the body is surrounded by a membrane that's made up of animal fats. When a person does not eat sufficient amounts of raw animal fat their cell membranes malfunction, resulting in diminished cellular nourishment and cleansing. Raw animal fats provide stable energy levels, and are required to heal the body. They also happen to be delicious, deeply satiating, and prevent sugar cravings.

Raw animal fats are mostly saturated, unlike fats from plants which are mostly unsaturated. It was previously thought that saturated fats were not good for heath, and unsaturated fats were beneficial. This simplistic perspective has proven to be hugely incorrect during the last two decades. Raw animals fats are especially good at lubricating the joints, building strong bones, dissolving arterial plaque, enhancing immunity, and moisturizing the skin.

Raw animal fats feed the brain and nervous system; two organs that are starving and toxic in the modern world. Since the brain is composed of 60% fat, when you eat raw animal fats you are literally feeding your brain the raw materials that it requires. The brain is usually starving and therefore malfunctioning in people who don't eat enough fat. Symptoms of animal fat deficiency include memory problems, brain fog, spaciness, anxiety, multiple-sclerosis, Parkinson's, and even Alzheimer's.

Raw animal fats are also essential in creating a healthy pregnancy, and are ideally eaten for several years prior to pregnancy and also during pregnancy. This practice will nourish, protect, and cleanse mother and baby. To heighten fertility levels prior to conception traditional cultures ate raw butter, and in fact prized it as a sacred fertility food. Raw animal fats will also support the manufacture and balance of hormones before, during, and after pregnancy. If you have any fertility concerns please consider not placing a laptop computer on your lap. This is a very effective way to sterilize yourself.

In a toxic laden world people who are deficient in raw animal fats become more vulnerable to the detrimental effect of toxins. This is because raw animal fat (not cooked fat) surrounds each cell and acts as a protective barrier that prevents toxins from entering the cell. My personal experience has shown that raw fats cleanse my body extremely well. It's been shown that disease is largely the result of cellular toxic waste that has not been removed. Raw fats, especially animal fats, bind to toxic matter and carry it out of the body through the stool. These wonderful raw animal fats also cleanse and protect the liver.

> ~ *Raw animal fat (not cooked fat) surrounds each cell*
> *and acts as a protective barrier that prevents*
> *toxins from entering the cell.* ~

Fat-Soluble Vitamins

One thing I like about raw animal fats is that they are loaded with the critical fat-soluble vitamins A, D, E, and K2. These vitamins are found in high amounts in raw eggs, raw butter, and raw liver. These essential vitamins function synergistically and help to absorb a lot of other nutrients. Dr. Weston A. Price referred to these fat-soluble vitamins as "activators" because they help to absorb minerals. This is why when I occasionally cook veggies I smother them in raw butter after they've been cooked.

True vitamin A is fat-soluble, and is sometimes confused with beta-carotene which is a precursor of vitamin A. True vitamin A is only found in animal foods while beta-carotene is only found in plant foods. The body can convert precursor beta-carotene to true vitamin A, however in some people this ability is limited. Luckily raw butter, raw eggs, and raw liver contain high amounts of true vitamin A which absorbs very easily in the body.

Fat-soluble vitamin A is known to promote beautiful skin, protect against infections, produce sex hormones, promote healthy thyroid function, and enhance eyesight. I've noticed that my night vision is so much better since eating foods that are rich in vitamin A. This crucial vitamin is used up in the presence of stress, fever, and heavy exercise. Vitamin A needs to be adequately replaced during these periods.

Fat-soluble vitamin D is one of the most common nutrient deficiencies. When people are deficient in vitamin D they exhibit a long list of diseases such as cancer, depression, osteoporosis, asthma, cardiovascular disease, diabetes, autoimmune disorders, brain problems, and infections. Exposure to regular sunshine, and adequate consumption of raw butter, raw eggs, and raw liver, ensure that you will have sufficient amounts of this critical nutrient.

Fat-soluble vitamin E is a potent antioxidant that protects cells from the damaging effects of free radicals. It relies on dietary fat for proper absorption. Vitamin E is involved in many processes such as immune function, formation of red blood cells, cleansing the arteries, reducing scarring, vasodilation, promotion of supple skin, thinning the blood, and increasing endurance.

Another fat-soluble vitamin is vitamin K2. This vitamin is found in high amounts during the summer months when grass-fed milk, butter, and cheese have a deep yellow color. Vitamin K2 cleans plaque from the arteries, is required for strong bones, promotes growth, and activates cellular repair. For anyone concerned with osteoporosis it's good to know vitamin K2 and vitamin D are synergistic; they need each other to function better.

Five

Eat Fat to Lose Fat

I've been eating a high fat diet for several years and have experienced great results. I was especially inspired to eat a lot of raw fat after reading Sally Fallon's book *Eat Fat to Lose Fat*. I now tell people that I'm on the eat fat to lose fat diet. My understanding is that ancestrally, fat and protein were the most available foods. This tells me that nature intended for people to eat a diet that's high in raw healthy fats. When you're not eating enough healthy raw fats your body will tend to store fat because fat is needed for the maintenance of health. Eating the right kinds of fats tells the body that food is abundant, which in turn allows the body to release stored fat.

When you consume sufficient amounts of raw fats you may notice that you're able to go for hours without food cravings. This happens because your blood sugar has been stabilized. Eating raw fats is like giving your body an "oil change," because as the new healthy fats are eaten the old unhealthy stored fats are released. Your car runs more smoothly and efficiently after an oil change, and so will you.

One of the reasons why I like a diet that's high in raw fat is because after my raw egg and raw butter smoothies I feel deeply satiated without gaining weight. Recently a friend asked me how I can eat so much raw fat and not gain weight even though I never count calories. Using his calorie counter he entered the food I had eaten during the day and to our surprise it only came to 1,200 calories, which is really not a lot of calories. The calories from raw foods are truly satiating, that's why you don't need to eat a lot of food when you eat raw paleo.

~ *Remember to eat for quality not quantity.* ~

Raw paleo gives me the nutrition I need without any unnecessary snacking. Eating small amounts of raw nutrient-dense whole foods is the key. Remember to eat for quality not quantity.

Six

FRIENDLY CHOLESTEROL

Cholesterol has been erroneously seen as the bad guy for far too long. Like everyone, I used to think cholesterol clogged arteries, caused heart disease, and made you fat. However, once I began my personal research I discovered the truth about cholesterol. I realized that it's an essential lipid, our friend, and is even produced by our body on a daily basis. So why do so many people believe that it's harmful?

Foods that contain cholesterol such as eggs, butter, and animal meats have been given a bad rap during the last several decades, however it's only because cholesterol has been grossly misunderstood. Increasingly more studies show no relationship between diet and cholesterol levels. (7) In fact, as Americans have cut back on saturated fats and cholesterol heart disease has actually increased. (8) There is no evidence that saturated fats and cholesterol-rich foods contribute to heart disease!

Many factors are known to contribute to heart disease. These include oxidized cholesterol from heated cooking oils, sugar, toxins, lack of collagen-forming nutrients, trans fats, inactivity, and poor sleep. The reality is that many factors contribute to heart disease, and cholesterol is not one of them. (9) Blaming cholesterol in food for cardiovascular disease lacks both scientific and real life evidence.

Cholesterol, in fact, plays an important role in preventing cardiovascular disease due to its ability to "patch" the walls of weakened blood vessels. Without this essential patch the weakened blood vessel walls would rupture causing hemorrhages, aneurisms, and other problems associated with broken blood vessels. Cholesterol is really your friend and a lifesaver.

The body cannot function properly without cholesterol. This essential lipid is actually contained in every cell of the body. Cholesterol forms a vital part of cell membranes, which serve to protect cells from invading toxins. When the body is deficient in cholesterol toxins are able to easily enter the cells, causing a myriad of diseases.

Without adequate amounts of cholesterol the brain and nervous system cannot function correctly. Recent research has shown that elderly people with higher cholesterol levels have better memory than those with lower levels. Research from the Norwegian University of Science and Technology showed that woman with high cholesterol levels live longer than woman with low cholesterol. (10) Several cohort studies of healthy people show that low cholesterol levels are also a risk factor for cancer. So feel free to eat all the raw cholesterol that your body desires.

~ *Cholesterol helps to balance your hormones.* ~

Cholesterol also helps to balance your hormones, which in turn helps to normalize many bodily functions. You'll feel more calm, happy, and healthy by eating raw cholesterol. As of this writing, the US government has now officially removed cholesterol from the list of bad foods. Eating cholesterol is now considered a healthful act, and there are no limitations on quantity.

Hormones Synthesized from Cholesterol

ESTROGEN
Estrogen is required for building bones, brain health, and normal reproductive processes.

PROGESTERONE
Progesterone plays and important role in sex hormone production, brain function, regulation of menstrual cycles, supporting the early stages of pregnancy, and promotion of healthful gestation. Progesterone also relieves the symptoms of menopause.

ALDOSTERONE
Regulates electrolytes, and prevents water retention.

DHEA
Improves memory, immunity, bone density, and adrenal function. Since DHEA functions like a growth hormone it has anti-aging properties, such as the ability to increase muscle mass. It also reduces wrinkles, hair loss, and dryness of skin.

TESTOSTERONE
Helps libido, vitality, strength, and improves youthfulness.

CORTISOL
Cortisol is an adrenal hormone that regulates inflammation, balances the immune system, and stabilizes blood pressure. When produced at the right times and the right amounts cortisol helps us to sleep better at night.

Vᴛᴀᴍɪɴ **D**
Is involved with the immune system, calcium absorption, cancer protec-
tion, healthy nervous system, mineral absorption, muscle tone, insulin
stabilization, and fertility.

Cholesterol helps to improve levels of vitamin D, a deficiency that's
become epidemic in America. When you eat sufficient amounts of raw
cholesterol you will also have optimal quantities of cholesterol on your
skin, which helps you absorb vitamin D from sunlight. So next time you're
sunbathing you can rest assured that your skin has enough cholesterol to
manufacture vitamin D.

Cholesterol gives you smooth and glowing skin because it allows your
skin to hold onto the right amount of water. Remember, it's not only how
much water you drink but also how much moisture is held in your skin.
Cholesterol also helps the skin by repairing damaged skin cells.

~ *Moisture is held in your skin by cholesterol.* ~

Unbeknownst to many people, cholesterol is the unsung antioxidant. It
protects you from free radicals and their oxidizing effects. Yes, that's right,
cholesterol is anti-aging!

Consuming liberal amounts of raw cholestcrol can be highly beneficial
for people of all ages. My friend, a 70 year old male, has been on the raw
paleo diet for 15 years. He has a super vital sex life which he attributes to
the large amounts of raw cholesterol that he eats. His favorite cholesterol-
rich foods are raw eggs, raw butter, and raw cream. The liver produces approximately 75% of the cholesterol that the body requires. However, the

liver may be unable to produce sufficient amounts of cholesterol when it's burdened with excessive toxins found in food, air, water, and pharmaceuticals. This problem may be further exacerbated in people who consume alcohol. In these instances, the body's cholesterol production may have to be augmented by eating raw cholesterol.

TIDBITS ON CHOLESTEROL

Cholesterol powers the entire body by transmitting signals from the brain to all of the glands and organs. Therefore, low cholesterol equates to glands and organs that function below par.

Cholesterol is used by the liver to produce bile acids, which help you to digest and absorb fats and fat-soluble vitamins. When fat cannot be digested and absorbed, the body stores it as adipose tissue. Yes, a deficiency of cholesterol can make you fat. Wrinkles also form due to a lack of lubrication in the skin. Wrinkled and obese is not my idea of sexy!

~ A deficiency of cholesterol can make you fat. ~

People with low cholesterol levels are known to be depressed and aggressive. This is because serotonin receptors use cholesterol in order to release the "feel good" hormones. Raw eggs, which are rich in cholesterol, are known to help calm aggressive dogs.

Breast milk is high in cholesterol which is required for proper growth, brain development, and immune function of the baby. Cholesterol helps to maintain cell integrity through out the entire body, including the intestines. Low cholesterol diets can lead to leaky gut and other digestive disorders.

Seven

FRESH ORGANIC RAW PROTEIN

Protein has been a hot topic ever since my raw vegan days. During that period I was led to believe that we don't need a lot of protein, and that animal protein creates cancer and many other diseases. Back then I started noticing that I was losing muscle mass, was always hungry, my hair was thinning, and my bones felt weak. I was also concerned because my recovery after bodily injuries was much longer than before. However, I was repeatedly told that plant protein is better than animal protein. How could this be, especially with the new symptoms I was experiencing?

Protein is a macronutrient that's necessary for the proper growth of nerves, glands, organs, muscles, and other protein derived body parts. Protein from animal meats is similar to the protein of our body, and can therefore be used more easily than its vegan counterpart. Protein, like fat, satiates the appetite and helps to maintain body weight. Because I now eat raw animal protein, I am no longer constantly hungry.

Raw Paleo

The raw paleo way of eating focuses on <u>quality</u> not quantity. This is because raw proteins that have not been denatured by heat are more bioavailable and utilizable in the body. Many mainstream nutritionists instruct their clients to eat large quantities of cooked or powdered protein in order to correct certain ailments. However, large amounts of denatured protein cannot do what small quantities of raw protein are able to do in the body.

~ Raw protein is easy to digest
and does not impose a load on the kidneys. ~

I've noticed that when I eat <u>raw</u> protein I require a smaller amount than when I eat cooked protein. Raw protein is easy to digest and does not impose a load on the kidneys, unlike cooked protein which is more difficult to digest and imposes a greater load on the kidneys. Eating less raw protein also reduces the unnecessary killing of animals.

Eight

ORGANIC GRASS-FED RAW MILK

"The land of (raw) milk and (raw) honey"
Exodus 33.3 - The Holy Bible

One of my biggest health discoveries was when I first found out about raw milk. One day while exploring small towns in southern California my mother and I found a raw goat milk farm. We were so excited while chugging the raw milk that suddenly we realized how much our bodies were starving for this much-needed nutrition. We couldn't stop drinking it. We were looking at each other in awe and raising our glasses to cheers. It tasted great and we could feel how it was nourishing our bodies.

I didn't drink pasteurized milk while growing up, and thank God because it would have been factory farmed junk milk anyway. Most commercially available milk is from cows that are subjected to unhealthy and cruel conditions, and inappropriate feed that's laden with chemicals, antibiotics, and hormones. This junk milk is further degraded by pasteurization, homogenization, and standardization. This kind of milk does not do a body good.

The pasteurization of milk was conceived in the 1800's to supposedly kill "bad" bacteria, and to extend its shelf life. However, pasteurization of milk is a bad idea because it ruins the quality of the vitamins, minerals, proteins, fats, sugars, probiotics, enzymes, Life Force, and DNA of the milk. Killing microbes is unnecessary, unwise, and has many unwanted side-effects. (11) With pasteurization of milk come numerous health problems such as osteoporosis, tooth decay, diabetes, ear infections, allergies, autoimmune disease, and gastrointestinal aliments just to name a few.

The pasteurization of milk has continued because it allows the farmer to produce cheap milk. However, this milk is contaminated with illness-causing pathogens due to the unsanitary farming conditions. Pasteurization is definitely required for this milk that's contaminated with pathogens, however due to pasteurization it cannot support health like its raw counterpart.

Note: When you buy any drink such as vegetable juice, coconut water, and fruit juice, you must look for unpasteurized, raw, and non-high pressure processing (HPP) products. HPP products are not truly raw.

If pasteurizations' devastating health effects don't make your blood boil then homogenizations' ill effects may. It might sound crazy but homogenization is only done for monetary reasons. This unnatural process splits the fat molecules into tiny pieces, thus allowing the fat to spread evenly throughout the milk. (12) The cream cannot separate and rise to the top of the bottle anymore, thereby greatly extending shelf life.

Similar to pasteurization, homogenization has devastating effects on health. When the process of homogenization was introduced, artery damage and heart disease started increasing. Lipid researcher, Mary Enig, PhD, claims that the artificial fat globules formed during homogenization clog the arteries which then reduces blood flow, nourishment, and oxygen to the heart. (13) Atherosclerosis and other cardiovascular diseases soon follow.

~ *Raw milk that comes straight from the cow is a superfood,*
unlike its pseudo counterpart. ~

Raw grass-fed milk is completely different to the pasteurized, homogenized, and standardized white liquid that is commonly sold under the guise of milk. What makes denatured milk even more of a problem are the added artificial vitamins such as calcium and vitamin D. As of this writing, the FDA has allowed this "white liquid" to become even more toxic through the addition of the artificial sweetener aspartame - yes, you read this correctly. Raw milk that comes straight from the cow is a superfood, unlike its pseudo counterpart.

Nutrients in Raw Milk

Amino Acids
Contains all of the 20 amino acids required for optimal health. This includes an impressive nine of the ten essential amino acids that the body cannot make and therefore has to get from food.

Omega 3 Polyunsaturated Fat
Contains an omega 3 fat called docosahexaenoic acid (DHA), which is extremely deficient in the standard American diet. DHA is only present

when animals are grass-fed. The brain and nervous system require large amounts of this nutrient in order to function correctly. Inflammation, which is epidemic nowadays, drops considerably when DHA levels are adequate.

OMEGA 6 POLYUNSATURATED FAT
Contains conjugated linoleic acid (CLA), which is extremely deficient in the standard American diet. CLA is only present when animals are grass-fed. CLA balances metabolism, promotes muscle growth, reduces insulin resistance, builds immunity, alleviates food allergies, protects against cancer, and decreases belly fat.

OMEGA 9 MONOUNSATURATED FAT
Contains oleic acid (OA), which helps to improve insulin sensitivity, blood circulation, and the regeneration of brain myelin.

SATURATED FATS
Contains an abundance of healthful saturated fats such as myristic acid, palmitic acid, and stearic acid.

ENZYMES
Contains 60 enzymes which help you digest all the nutrients found in milk. These enzymes aid metabolic processes in the body, and help prevent the growth of any possible bad microbes.

MINERALS
Contains 24 minerals, including the four major electrolytes calcium, potassium, magnesium, and sodium. Other important minerals are phosphorus, sulfur, boron, bromine, chromium, copper, iodine, nickel, vanadium, silica, chloride, fluoride, strontium, selenium, zinc, molybdenum, manganese, cobalt, tin, and iron.

FAT-SOLUBLE VITAMINS
Contains the fat-soluble vitamins A, D, E, and K2.

WATER-SOLUBLE VITAMINS
Contains the water-soluble B vitamins such as B1 (thiamine), B2 (riboflavin), vitamin B3 (niacin), B5 (pantothenate), B6 (pyridoxine), B9 (folate), B12 (cyanocobalamin), and biotin. Milk also contains vitamin C, which is only found in raw milk. The heat from the pasteurization process destroys this vitamin.

PROBIOTICS:
Contains beneficial bacteria which help to restore your gut microbiome, thereby improving immunity, brain function, and overall health.

PHOSPHATASE
Contains the enzyme phosphatase, which helps the body to absorb the calcium in the milk. This useful enzyme is heat labile, and therefore is missing in pasteurized milk. This is one of the many reasons why pasteurized milk contributes to the formation of osteoporosis.

THE MIRACLE OF RAW MILK
My friend Susan had been dealing with aching teeth that had black spots on them. I suggested she give raw milk a try. To her surprise, after just one month of drinking raw milk the toothaches and black spots disappeared. In my understanding, Susan's dental transformation is due to the highly bioavailable calcium, phosphorus, potassium, magnesium, enzymes, and possibly other nutrients found in raw milk. The black spots may have also been removed by the vitamin K2 in the raw milk which is known to remove plaque.

DIGESTIBILITY OF RAW MILK

When nature's foods are denatured the body oftentimes rejects them through allergies, sensitivities, and intolerances. This is especially true when raw milk is denatured. For example, some people are intolerant to the lactose (milk sugar) in pasteurized milk; they cannot digest the milk sugar. Maldigestion occurs because pasteurization has deactivated the inherent lactase enzyme which breaks down the milk sugar. (14) Your body is therefore pasteurization intolerant, which is different from true lactose intolerance. If your body can't handle the lactose in pasteurized milk then I suggest you give raw milk a try. If you're highly intolerant I recommend you start with a teaspoon of raw milk per day and increase slowly from there.

Some people may also experience digestive difficulties when drinking cold raw milk, therefore I don't recommend this. Raw milk is more easily digestible and assimilable when drunk at room temperature. Simply place the milk in a glass container, with a loose lid, into a cupboard for several hours or more. To enhance digestibility you can add raw honey to it before placing it in the cupboard.

To enhance digestibility even further you can make clabber, a kefir-like drink. Simply take a quart of raw milk, add one tablespoon of raw honey, place a loose lid on top, and put in a dark cupboard for 24-48 hours. Afterwards place the clabber in the refrigerator.

If you would like to occasionally drink cold raw milk I suggest you first hold it in your mouth until it's warm, and then swallow it. Remember to sip your milk, or any other liquid, and never gulp it down. Staying relaxed while eating will greatly help with the digestion of your food. If you're still experiencing uncomfortable symptoms, then you may want to find out the type of cow that produces your milk.

Another factor that contributes to the digestibility of raw milk is the type of cow that produced it. Cows are divided into two types: the newer breeds (A1) and the heritage breeds (A2). Newer cows such as Holsteins and Friesians produce more milk, however it's less nutritious and not as tasty. On the other hand, heritage cows produce less milk that's more nutritious and tastier. These cows include Jersey, Guernsey, Swiss, Normande, Asian, and African breeds. A2 heritage cows produce the original healthful milk.

However, A1 milk from the newer breeds can cause health problems. This milk usually contains a protein (beta casein) that is inflammatory for some people, and can cause eczema, allergies, heat disease, asthma, diabetes, autism, schizophrenia, auto-immune disease, mucus, and upper respiratory infections. If you're experiencing any of these symptoms after drinking raw milk, I suggest you check the type of cow your milk comes from.

Raw Milk Cheese

Raw whole milk cheese is a nutrient-dense food due to its high amount of protein, fat, and micronutrients. I sometimes like to eat raw cheese when I'm very hungry because it's deeply nourishing and satisfying. The good thing about raw cheese is that it's a complete meal.

Raw cheese has five times more calcium than raw milk, and therefore is great for restoring a calcium deficiency. Common calcium deficiencies include cavities, osteoporosis, receding gums, muscle spasms, high blood pressure, and anxiety. To absorb more minerals from the raw cheese you can spread raw honey on it.

~ *Raw cheese has five times more calcium than raw milk.* ~

One of the lesser know functions of raw cheese is its powerful ability to soak up toxins. When you're feeling nauseous, a sign that toxins are in the stomach, eating a cube of raw cheese will help to absorb the toxins and escort them out of the body. Raw cheese has helped me many times in removing toxins from my stomach.

Due to its toxin-soaking ability some people may become constipated when eating raw cheese. To lessen the possibility of constipation, make sure that your raw cheese contains <u>sea</u> salt. Spreading raw butter on the raw cheese also reduces the chance of constipation.

Eating a small cube of raw whole milk cheese throughout the day can help stabilize your blood sugar level. This stabilizing effect is due to the high amount of fat and protein in the raw cheese. Simply place several small cubes of raw cheese in a 4oz glass jar, and take with you during the day.

<u>Note</u>: Much of the raw cheese you purchase in US markets is not truly raw. Many US manufacturers heat their cheese to one degree below pasteurization. This cheese is legally still considered raw, however is technically pasteurized. To make sure you're getting truly raw cheese, I recommend buying imported raw cheese from Europe, Organic Pastures' raw cheese from California, and raw cheese from small local farmers.

Nine

ORGANIC GRASS-FED RAW BUTTER

If heaven were a food it would be raw butter.

One of my favorite foods is raw butter. My eyes are delighted by its rich yellow color, the taste is creamy and delicious, and my body feels deeply satiated. Cows that graze on green pasture produce a beautiful yellow butter that's highly nutritious. This nutritional delicacy is made from the cream which rises to the top of whole raw milk. The cream is then skimmed off and cold churned into butter.

Raw grass-fed butter is rich in saturated fats, omega 3 fats, and omega 6 fats. These fats are crucial for feeding the brain. Raw grass-fed butter is rich in the fat-soluble vitamins A, D, E, and K2. It also contains iodine, manganese, chromium, zinc, copper, and selenium. Raw butter has a myriad of nutrients that are easily absorbed due to the raw fats in the butter.

I'm happy to see that raw butter, a traditional food, has started to make a comeback at many family meals. Due to its content of saturated fat, raw butter was once wrongfully blamed as being the cause of high cholesterol, and resulting heart disease. We were told to eat margarine, vegetable oils, and low-fat foods which soon ushered in the low-fat diet era. People thought they were going to become healthier by eating this way, however the exact opposite happened. We saw a big increase in cardiovascular disease, multiple sclerosis, Alzheimer's, Parkinson's and many problems that still linger from this extremist unscientific era.

~ *Raw butter is a traditional staple.* ~

Decades of empirical evidence and updated science now show us that raw butter is not only safe to eat but *udderly* beneficial. It provides many health benefits such as strong bones, supple joints, healthy skin, supports the balancing of hormones, sustained energy levels, and proper brain function. When raw butter is grass-fed it has strong anticancer properties, is antimicrobial, and is full of probiotics especially when you eat the cultured version.

Due to the many healing properties of raw butter it has become a staple in my diet. Before starting to eating raw paleo I used to have some nagging conditions which were helped by the advice of a friend. He used to tell me to eat more raw butter no matter what the ailment was. He would lift the skin on my hand and say that I was dry. "You need to eat more raw butter because it keeps your skin supple," he would say. I'd mention to him that I was constipated and he'd remark "You need to eat more raw butter to lubricate your intestines." I'd tell him that I had cramps and he would repeat that I needed to eat more raw butter because it supports the balancing of hormones. When I felt anxious or ungrounded… yep… the same was true: eat more raw butter. I finally I got it. I needed to eat more raw butter! Now my favorite saying is "when in doubt eat more raw butter."

~ *Eat more raw butter!* ~

I'm happy with the wonderful health benefits raw butter has brought to my life. I started the raw paleo diet by eating one pound of grass-fed butter per week, but now that my cells are well fed I eat about 1/4 pound. Butter is truly a miraculous food.

Note: I do not recommend that beginners eat lots of raw butter due to the possibility of experiencing a Herxheimer reaction, which is an excessive and unnecessary cleansing response of the body. You can start out with one teaspoon and build from there.

Benefits of Raw Butter

THE BRAIN
The brain is made up predominantly of lipids: fat and cholesterol. Raw butter contains high amounts of saturated fat which nourish the brain. It also has an omega 6 fat called arachidonic acid (ARA), which also supports brain function and plays a vital role in the brain development of children. This is possibly why children like to eat so much butter. Grass-fed raw butter also contains an omega 6 fat called conjugated linoleic acid (CLA), which is protective to the brain especially in its anti-angiogenic properties.

Grass-fed raw butter contains good amounts of docosahexaenoic acid (DHA), which is one of the predominate fats in the brain. Recent research has shown that your body can synthesize DHA through curcumin found in turmeric, and boost levels of this fat in the brain. (15)   In fact, the body is able to synthesize DHA through several different mechanisms. You can make a raw butter turmeric spread that you can use in your raw paleo recipes. Raw butter is a super power food for your brain!

WEIGHT LOSS

Raw butter contains conjugated linoleic acid (CLA) which the body uses for fat loss and muscle building. Another reason why raw butter helps you to lose weight is because it has many nutrient-dense calories that decrease appetite and reduce cravings. What a nice fat!

SKIN, IMMUNITY, AND EYES

Vitamin A, D, and E found in raw butter are good for the skin, immune system, and eyes. Vitamin A, D, and E are effective at removing infections from the body. The scientific name for vitamin A is retinol, which is found in the retina of the eye. A mild deficiency of vitamin A causes night blindness. A severe deficiency can cause a detached retina, and in pregnant mothers can cause blindness in the baby.

THE THYROID GLAND

Raw butter contain four nutrients that are good for thyroid function: vitamin A, selenium, zinc, and iodine. The thyroid gland requires large amounts of vitamin A, and cannot function properly without it. This gland greatly influences emotional well being, so take good care of it.

FERTILITY AND GROWTH

Raw butter, with its high amounts of fat-soluble vitamins, is the perfect prenatal and postnatal food. Many indigenous cultures prized raw butter as a sacred food for fertility, reproduction, and reduction of pain during childbirth. Weston A. Price showed that when women ate a diet high in vitamin A, their children had broad faces, straight teeth, and well-formed bone structure. Raw butter gives you the extra fat-soluble nutrients that your body needs during and after pregnancy.

LUBRICATION OF JOINTS

Raw butter contains the *Wulzen Factor,* an anti-stiffness nutrient, which is <u>only</u> found in raw butter and raw cream. This is a hormone-like substance that helps to lubricate the joints, reduce joint calcification, and relieves arthritis. It also helps to prevent cataracts and pineal calcification. (16)   However, this unique nutrient is destroyed by pasteurization. When calves drink pasteurized milk they develop joint stiffness, but their symptoms are reversed when raw dairy fat is reintroduced into their diets. Go ahead, enjoy raw butter, and improve your joint mobility.

OSTEOPOROSIS

Raw butter is the perfect food to help with osteoporosis due to its fat-soluble vitamins A, D, E, and K2. The fat in butter supports the absorption of minerals that are required for building strong bones, such as calcium, magnesium, phosphorus, strontium, and silica. Raw butter is truly a magnificent support for healthy bones.

DIGESTION

Raw butter is great at healing the intestines. The primary fat in raw butter is butyric acid, a saturated short chain fatty acid, which supports the health of the intestinal wall. Nowadays butyric acid is used to treat inflammatory bowel disorders, such as Crohn's disease.

Raw butter also contains a complex lipid called glycosphingolipid which helps prevent gut infections. Eating liberal amounts of raw butter will lubricate your intestinal tract, and reduce intestinal infections and inflammation. I've personally noticed a great improvement in my overall digestion and previous constipation issues after eating raw butter.

ANTIOXIDANTS

Antioxidants serve many essential functions in the body because they scavenge free radicals. Without antioxidants, the process of disease and aging greatly accelerates. Raw butter contains antioxidants such as selenium, vitamin A, vitamin E, and cholesterol. Antioxidants are like a superhero at work in your body.

ANTIMICROBIAL

In this day and age of rampant infections raw butter is your protector and faithful friend. The short chain and medium chain saturated fatty acids found in raw butter are antibacterial, antiviral, and antifungal. Vitamin A, vitamin E, and selenium found in raw butter also help to reduce the incidence of infections. Raw butter is specifically great at preventing Candida overgrowth because it contains antifungal fats such as lauric acid, capric acid, and butyric acid. This is yet another important reason to eat raw butter.

A Note about Unhealthy Oils

There is much confusion in the area of oils. Some oils are healthy and others are outright toxic. The old paradigm that vegetable oils are healthy and animal fats (saturated) are detrimental lacks real life evidence. Several decades of empirical data, backed by modern science, has shown us that this simplistic view is incorrect.

Evidence over several decades has shown us that arteries are clogged by heated vegetable oils, trans fats, and any type of fat that has been denatured by homogenization, pasteurization, or other means. Even heated or dehydrated flax seeds may clog the arteries due to their high omega 3 content.

~ *Stay away from Canola!!!* ~

Oils that should <u>never</u> be consumed are canola, soybean, and cottonseed. Unhealthy oils cause inflammation, clogging of arteries, cellulite, skin outbreaks, lymphatic congestion, and many other problems. These unhealthy oils are foreign to the body and only came about during the last century. They provide very little nutrition and some even contain GMO's. Lastly, olive oil is predominantly an omega 9 fat which means that when it is heated it oxidizes and becomes toxic.

I personally like to avoid palm oil because even though it's healthy, commercial use of this oil has destroyed the forest habitat of the orangutan. When cooking, the best types of fat (not raw) are coconut oil, ghee, beef tallow, and pork lard.

Ten

Organic Pasture-Raised Raw Eggs

Did you know that raw eggs are the original superfood, especially when they're pasture-raised? These eggs are far superior to free-range, cage-free, and vegetarian-fed eggs, which is misleading hype that doesn't mean much. Many nutritional experts claim that raw eggs are nature's perfect health food. I especially like raw eggs because they make me feel so good, and are quick and easy to eat.

Pasture-raised eggs are eggs from chickens that live outdoors on grass all day long. A chicken raised on pasture will live a healthier life and produce eggs with superior nutritional content. Please do not eat conventionally raised eggs because they're produced from sick chickens, which produce unhealthy eggs.

Unlike common lore, chickens are omnivores and their natural diet is meant to be made up of larva, worms, bugs, seeds, grasses, roots, sunlight, and fresh air. If one day you get to raise your own chickens you'll find that they like to eat the pulp of freshly made vegetable juice, or any other food that you may compost. Raising backyard chickens is becoming increasingly popular in the USA.

Raw eggs contain macronutrients and micronutrients that are easily digestible and absorbable. The fat, protein, and numerous micronutrients can digest within 30 minutes when eaten raw. If you cook eggs they end up losing some of their inherent healing potential. Bodybuilders have known about the muscle building aspects of raw eggs and have eaten them for many decades. Raw eggs contain all 18 amino acids in a form that's highly bioavailable allowing the entire body, including muscles, to be easily nourished. I feel so good when I eat 1-2 raw eggs rocky style daily.

Some people are concerned about eating raw eggs because they've been told that the avidin in the egg white will deplete the biotin in their body. After doing much research I've come to understand that egg yolks are one of nature's richest sources of biotin. There is ample biotin in the yolk to counteract all of the avidin in the white. However, if you only eat egg whites, whether raw or cooked, the avidin in the whites will definitely deplete the biotin in your body. Recent research shows that even when egg whites are cooked, only a small percentage of the avidin is deactivated. I wonder if avidin's tolerance to heat may be because it's a required nutrient for the synergistic functioning of the other nutrients in the egg.

I have personally interviewed many people who have eaten raw eggs for several decades, and no one has ever had a biotin deficiency nor have they heard of anyone who has had a biotin deficiency. The more I've come to understand nature, the more I've realized that nature knows what its doing. Fragmentation or alteration of nature, in any way, is unwise.

The most nutrient-dense part of an egg is the yolk, however it's also the least understood. You can safely do away with the old myth that you're just supposed to eat the egg whites if you want to be fit and healthy. Eggs are meant to be eaten whole just the way nature made them. Cholesterol in raw egg yolks supports the synthesis and balancing of many hormones, including estrogen and progesterone. Raw eggs yolks are also good for fertility, female and male. Since I'm approaching my late thirties I eat raw eggs to keep my own eggs fertile.

The yolk of the egg is rich in two carotenoids: lutein and zeaxanthin. These two antioxidants help in the prevention of eye diseases such as macular degeneration, detached retina, and cataracts. Some people refer to lutein and zeaxanthin as the two superfoods that stop blindness. If eggs are cooked, the lutein and zeaxanthin are altered and therefore won't be absorbed as well.

Collagen will give you a natural "lift" in places where you need it most. The white portion of raw eggs is exceedingly high in utilizable collagen, which is required for youthful skin, healthy joints, lustrous hair, and strong nails. Sulfur, a precursor to collagen, is found abundantly in whole raw eggs. Raw whole eggs are a great anti-aging food due to their collagen properties.

Raw eggs are rich in the fat-soluble vitamins A, D, E, and K2. When pasture-raised they're also a great source of docosahexaenoic acid (DHA), an omega-3 fat. Eggs contain many B vitamins such as B1 (thiamin), B2 (riboflavin), B3 (niacin), B5 (pantothenate), B6 (pyridoxine), folate, biotin, and are especially rich in vitamin B12. Minerals found in raw eggs include calcium, magnesium, potassium, sodium, sulfur, chlorine, phosphorous, manganese, iodine, copper, iron, selenium, molybdenum, and zinc. An impressive list of minerals, I'd say.

Due to the high amounts of choline in raw eggs they can improve the functioning of your brain and nervous system. This nutrient is great for helping with brain fog and cognitive issues. Choline is a precursor to a neurotransmitter called acetylcholine, which is good for your heart and intestines. Choline can also powerfully cleanse your liver. Deficiencies cause various types of muscle problems, fatty liver disease, poor memory, kidney necrosis, and fatigue.

~ *Raw whole eggs are modern day heroes because they can rescue you from countless toxins.* ~

Raw whole eggs are modern day heroes because they can rescue you from countless toxins. They contain macro and micronutrients that help your body detoxify in four different ways. Firstly, the fat in the yolk is great at binding to petrochemically-based toxins, which constitute most of the current poisons on our planet. The fat in the yolk does this by binding to the toxins and carrying them out of the body through the stools.

Secondly, the protein in raw egg yolks and whites can bind to non-petrochemically-based toxins such as heavy metals. The bound heavy metals are then excreted via the stools. This detox pathway is yet another reason why it's best to eat your eggs in the raw.

Thirdly, raw eggs also detox the body through their many detoxification nutrients such as sulfur, magnesium, selenium, zinc, molybdenum, choline, B vitamins, and vitamin A.

The fourth way that raw eggs detoxify the body is through their complete amino acid profile, which supports phase one and phase two liver detoxification. The primary amino acids used in these pathways are glutamine and cysteine. These two amino acids are responsible for manufacturing glutathione, the master antioxidant in the liver.

When you're feeling unwell or are in need of detoxification, consider eating raw eggs even though many people don't think of raw eggs in this way. Raw eggs are one of the best foods for liver support, detoxification, and overall health. So make sure to add raw eggs to your smoothies!

Due to the high amounts of detoxifying nutrients found in raw eggs, I find that when I eat raw eggs alone I notice slight detoxification effects. However, when I eat them as a part of my raw paleo recipes I don't feel this effect. To detox your body I recommend that you eat raw eggs by themselves. If you're going to eat the raw eggs rocky style I suggest that you start with one raw egg per day and increase by one raw egg each successive week. As a rule women can build up to 3 raw eggs per day and men up to 4 daily.

Beware of Soy and Corn in Eggs

Most farmers use a supplemental feed for their chickens which can contain soy or corn. Oftentimes people think that they are allergic to eggs, however in many cases they are allergic to the soy or corn in the supplemental feed. When the soy or corn has additionally been genetically modified (GMO) the allergic reactions are intensified. Beware.... we end up eating what the chickens eat.

Make sure to ask your farmer if the supplemental feed is soy free and corn free. Remember that in nature the early bird catches the worm not the legume. Chickens need to eat protein from worms, bugs, and larvae.

What is Salmonella?

The salmonella family of bacteria contains approximately 2,300 strains that, just like all microbes, are beneficial and meant to support health. These bacteria reside naturally in the gut of animals and people. However, since the late 1970's salmonella has taken a turn for the worse; outbreaks have become increasingly more common. In my understanding there are two causes for this. The first contributing cause is that factory farming raises sick chickens. The second is the ever-increasing deficiency and imbalance in the gut microbiome of people, which makes them vulnerable to mutated salmonella and all other types of microbes.

Factory farms are the birthplace of salmonella due to their numerous practices that work against nature. These include filthy and overcrowded conditions, incorrect feed, antibiotics, chemicals, inhumane treatment, and a lack of sunlight. Salmonella outbreaks occur when the feces of sick chickens from factory farms find their way onto the meat, which is later eaten by people. (17), (18) This is bad enough for the average person, however, the problem worsens when a person with a compromised gut microbiome ingests these traces of feces.

~ *Salmonella contamination is the farmer's responsibility,*
not the chickens'. Don't blame the chickens. ~

The responsibility for salmonella poisoning is always given to the chicken, however the true responsibility lies with the factory farmers who raise the sick chickens. Salmonella contamination is the farmer's responsibility, not the chickens'. Don't blame the chickens. The chance of salmonella outbreaks occurring in healthfully raised organic chickens is extremely low. Healthy chickens produce healthy food. Sick chickens produce sick food. When we mess with any natural process, we ultimately pay the price. It's that simple.

How to Buy Healthy Eggs

When you purchase eggs directly from a small farmer they will sometimes be underwashed and will have a natural coating on them called bloom. The bloom is a natural protective layer that seals the shell's pores and protects it from any invading bacteria. Commercially raised are washed in chemicals that remove this protective bloom. Mineral oil is then applied in order to replace the natural bloom. It is the mineral oil that makes store bought eggs shine.

It's unwise to remove nature's healthful coating and replace it with toxic mineral oil. Unfortunately, denaturing nature is a reoccurring pattern in modern nature-disconnected societies. Unlike washed eggs, fresh underwashed eggs can sit on your counter for weeks without spoiling.

<u>**Make sure that your raw eggs are always ORGANIC and PASTURE-RAISED.**</u>

Eleven

FRESH ORGANIC GRASS-FED RAW MEAT

My first bite of raw meat was at Rawesome, a private food buying club in Venice, California. One of the workers at Rawesome had prepared a raw meat dish for me called steak tartare. Even as a hardcore vegan, after eating it I lived through it. It was tasty and no big deal. My body gave me a definite yes! I've been enjoying raw meat ever since that first bite.

Raw meat is actually eaten in many parts of the world. Examples are carpaccio in Italy, steak tartare in France, and kibbeh in the Middle East and North Africa. The Japanese also have their version of a raw meat dish. I'm always fascinated as to why raw meat dishes are only available in exclusive restaurants. I don't cook my fruit, so why would I choose to cook my meat? They are both living foods; let's not kill our food.

~ *Raw meat is eaten in many parts of the world.* ~

Organic Grass-Fed Beef

There are two methods of raising cattle. One is where the cattle graze freely on grasslands, and is known as grass-fed meat. The other is where the cattle are confined to overcrowded barns and is referred to as factory farming or Confined Animal Feeding Operations (CAFO). When eating raw meat it's important to know how your food was raised.

Raising cattle organically and grass-fed is the best method of farming because it yields healthy meat, restores grasslands, and is good for the environment unlike conventional farming. Cattle are raised on a natural diet of perennial grasses, and herds are continually rotated on the fields. After the cattle have grazed and fertilized the soil, the grass is then given a chance to restore itself and become grassland once again for the next feeding. Grass-fed animals are good at fertilizing the soil; they feed themselves while simultaneously spreading their own manure. This saves on the use of synthetic fertilizers that are used in factory farming. Additionally, grass-fed farming does away with the fossil fuel that otherwise would have been used to transport the cattle's feed to the feedlots.

Studies have shown that when cattle are raised organically and grass-fed, their meat and other products have a greater nutritional profile. According to Michael Pollan and other experts, cows are designed to eat grass and cannot digest grains of any kind, including soy and corn. (19) They actually get sick when they eat grains. Grass-fed meat is much higher in nutrients including omega-3 fats, vitamin E, and CLA (conjugated linoleic acid). CLA is an important fat that's known to reduce the risk of cancer, diabetes, and immune system disorders.

~ *Grass-fed meat is much higher in nutrients.* ~

On the other hand, conventional factory farming poisons the soil and therefore the water substrates. It also depletes the soil of its minerals and microorganisms. Animals are fed an unnatural and chemicalized diet of corn, soybeans, grains, and other foreign feed. Conventional factory farming requires that grains are grown on an excessively large scale to specifically feed the cattle. The animals are fed incorrect toxic food, and the land is poisoned and depleted. Not a recipe for sustainability.

Conventional farming uses numerous poisons. These include fertilizers, pesticides, herbicides, fungicides, insecticides, miticides, rodenticides, bactericides, nematicides, and termiticides. These poisons seep into the ground and pollute all of our waters: aquifers, lakes, streams, and oceans. This harms aquatic life and the people who drink the water. The poisons that are sprayed also rise up into the air, adding to the already excessive carbon footprint. Each year our food, water, and air are increasingly poisoned, making health more difficult to attain each successive year.

Another problem with factory farming is that the animals are kept in stressful environments where they are packed tightly together in dirty conditions. Imagine standing in a phone booth with three other people who are pooping and peeing... and there's no way out? These stinky unhygienic conditions are the perfect breeding ground for deadly germs such as <u>mutated</u> strains of e-coli, which makes cattle sick and kills many Americans each year. Sick animals require large doses of antibiotics which masks their symptoms, but they're still sick. Sick animals in turn make the people who eat their meat sick! In an attempt to remove the overgrowth of mutated microbes from the filthy and sick meat, agribusiness then irradiates the meat. Irradiation is a form of gamma radiation which depletes many nutrients in the meat, forms new toxins in the meat, and makes this already toxic meat more harmful to eat.

The good news is that grass-fed meat is actually healthy for animals, people, and the planet. You can truly enjoy grass-fed meat and know that you're contributing to your health and planetary sustainability. By choosing organic grass-fed meat you're also reducing the demand for destructive factory farming.

For nutrition and safety reasons make sure that your meat is always ORGANIC, GRASS-FED and GRASS-FINISHED.

Note: Be cautious of the many labels that are used to confuse the novice consumer into believing that meat is grass-fed and grass-finished. I suggest you do not buy any meat unless it's clearly labeled as grass-fed and grass-finished.

THE HEALTH BENEFITS OF RAW MEAT

I remember being intrigued by how good I felt after first eating raw meat. It was afterwards that I learned about the vast array of nutrients found in raw meat. These life-giving nutrients explained why I felt so energized and calm every time I ate it. Even nowadays, whenever I eat raw meat I still feel as if I'm putting much needed nutrients into my body. It gives me a great energy boost, I no longer bruise the way I use to, and thankfully I never feel the urge to overeat. Raw meat is my vitamin supplement!

Raw meat may also be the ultimate anti-aging food. It contains all of the amino acids (building blocks) in a highly utilizable form, unlike the amino acids found in cooked meat. When you eat raw meat it's easily incorporated into human tissue and as such can regenerate collagen. Due to its blood stem cells, it can easily renew tissue cells. This muscle protein is obviously also great at building your own muscle tissue. Raw meat is chockfull of vitamins, minerals, antioxidants, enzymes, phospholipids, and healthy fats, which are responsible for meat's healing qualities.

~ *Raw meat may also be the ultimate anti-aging food.* ~

Another reason why I greatly appreciate eating raw meat is because it digests so easily, due to its full compliment of inherent enzymes. Many people know that vegetables contain enzymes, but did you know that raw meat and all raw animal foods also have an abundance of enzymes?

Raw meat is also a rich source of antioxidants, which are in dire need nowadays. These include glutathione, carnosine, conjugated linoleic acid (CLA), selenium, zinc, and iron. Raw meat is far more beneficial than many people believe.

Nutrients in Raw Meat
Raw meat contains all of the B vitamins, is one of the richest sources of vitamin B12, and has good amounts of niacin (vitamin B3), pantothenate (vitamin B5), pyridoxine (vitamin B6), and choline. It also contains some thiamine (vitamin B1) and folate (vitamin B9). These B vitamins are good for the nervous system, anemia, stress management, energy levels, hair, skin, and nails.

Raw meat contains high amounts of the minerals selenium, zinc, phosphorous, potassium, and iron. It also contains some magnesium, calcium, manganese, copper, and sodium. Since our soils are depleted of minerals this is another way to get these much needed minerals into your body.

Selenium is a wonderful anti-aging nutrient due to its powerful antioxidant function in the body. Selenium is the primary mineral used by the immune system. When this mineral is deficient all kinds of immune system problems and cancers can develop. Selenium is also used by the thyroid gland to stay healthy. It also protects against radiation and helps with fertility.

Zinc is so important to the body that it's used in over 200 enzymatic reactions. Every cell in the body relies on zinc for structure and function. A zinc deficiency may cause acne, hair loss, prostate problems, rashes, brain imbalances, nervous system issues, learning disabilities, and mental retardation. Zinc is especially important for wound healing, immunity, and warding off infections.

Potassium is an essential electrolyte that's required for proper contraction of muscles, including the heart muscle. It also helps to lower blood pressure; so yes, raw organic grass-fed meat is good for your heart. When potassium is in short supply you can also become confused, fatigued, or irritable. Potassium is also required to help you stay calm, and it does this by relaxing your nervous system.

~ *Raw organic grass-fed meat is good for your heart.* ~

The iron in raw meat is in the form of heme iron, which is a highly absorbable form of iron. Iron deficiency anemia can be easily treated with raw meat. Deficiencies can lead to oxygen reduction in tissues, balding, heart palpitations, learning difficulties, cracked lips and tongue, indecisiveness, and unassertiveness.

The fat-soluble vitamins A, D, E, and K2 are found in appreciable amounts in grass-fed beef. The marvel of nature forms these nutrients naturally in grass-fed, sunlight-absorbing animals. However, in grain-fed animals these nutrients are minimal.

Omega 3 fatty acids are found in good amounts in raw grass-fed meat, but not in grain-fed meat. Be aware of the fact that omega 3 fats are heat labile. This means that they are heat-sensitive and will oxidize when the meat is heated; they become toxic and unabsorbable to your body. This is yet another reason why it's best to eat grass-fed meat raw. Deficiencies of omega 3 fats include health problems such as inflammation, heart disease, memory problems, depression, attention deficit disorder, bipolar disorder, dry skin, brittle hair, hair loss, dandruff, and fatigue.

Conjugated linoleic acid (CLA) is also found in raw grass-fed meat. CLA is an omega 6 fatty acid that's present in grass-fed animals, but is non-existent when cows eat grain. CLA is known for its strong anti-cancer properties and has been shown to reduce tumors. CLA decreases body fat, increases muscle mass, improves immunity, and reduces bone loss.

Raw grass-fed meat also contains high amounts of a nutrient called CoQ10. This powerful antioxidant is good for heart health, cancer prevention, immunity, energy, and fertility. It's great at supporting the rejuvenation process and increasing longevity.

Due to the presence of glutamic acid, cysteine, and glycine raw meat helps the body manufacture a very important amino acid called glutathione. This amino acid is one of the most powerful antioxidants made by the body. Glutathione helps the liver to neutralize toxins, remove free radicals from the body, and generally helps you to detoxify. This antioxidant protects you from oxidative stress, illness, and aging. Raw meat also produces glutathione through alpha lipoic acid found in raw meat.

Please note that glutathione supplements cannot compare to raw meat, in terms of efficacy in the body. Supplements are isolates and do not contain the essential synergistic co-nutrients that are found in whole raw foods. Nutrients from food do not have toxic side effects as found with artificial, laboratory-made nutrients that are foreign to the body.

Raw meat also contains two unique amino acids, carnitine and carnosine, which are generally found in animal foods but are especially high in raw meat. These two nutrients have antioxidant functions, especially carnosine which is known for its anti-aging properties. These two amino acids have some overlapping functions in the body. The body can manufacture carnitine from lysine, vitamin B1, vitamin B6, and iron, however only when the liver is healthy.

Another important nutrient that's found only in meat is the amino acid creatine. This amino acid builds muscle and improves muscular endurance. It supplies energy to all cells thereby helping endurance athletes to train harder. Not only does creatine enhance athletic performance, it's also excellent for muscle recovery. Creatine helps with brain function, depression, muscular dystrophy, and chronic obstructive pulmonary disease (COPD).

Note: Some amino acids are sensitive to heat which means that cooking will alter and/or destroy some of these valuable amino acids.

Concerns about Bacteria in Raw Organic Grass-fed Meat

I'm oftentimes asked "How safe is the bacteria in raw meat?" I tell people I'm not afraid of bacteria in meat for two reasons. Firstly, the meat I eat is organic and grass-fed, and since bad bacteria have only been found in conventional farmed meat, I feel safe. Secondly, since people have a 10 to 1 ratio of bacteria to human cells, I realize that people are really bacteria sapiens! Our bodies are mostly microbes, so there's no need to fear ourselves.

> ~ *Our bodies are mostly microbes, so there's*
> *no need to fear ourselves.* ~

Humans are dependent on bacteria because they help us digest food, manufacture certain nutrients, and help other nutrients to be assimilated. Bacteria are also the natural garbage men of the body and help to consume diseased and dead cells. What would happen if the garbage men never showed up at your house? Your home would be filthy and stinky, wouldn't it? Many people's bodies have a similar problem. Therefore, embrace bacteria and they'll do their job of cleansing your body.

CONCERNS ABOUT PARASITES IN RAW ORGANIC GRASS-FED MEAT

I am not concerned about parasites because I always source clean and healthy meat. I've eaten raw paleo for five years and have never noticed any parasitic problems in clients, friends, or myself. I've even gone as far as interviewing dozens of people who've eaten raw meat for as long as 35 years and no one has ever experienced problems with parasites. They've also never heard of anyone who's experienced such problems.

When animals are raised correctly their meat or products do not contain harmful parasites. In order for meat to be parasite-free the animals must be raised organically, graze on open pastures, and be treated humanely. The meats or products of these healthy animals only contain microbes that are beneficial to people.

~ *Just like all microbes, parasites have a symbiotic relationship in the body.* ~

The body requires a certain amount of parasites in order to function healthfully. Just like all microbes, parasites have a symbiotic relationship in the body. Parasites may spawn as microscopic organisms or as macroscopic worms when needed. The microscopic organisms eat small toxic matter and the macroscopic worms eat larger toxic Matter. Toxic matter in the body results from an excessively high <u>toxic load</u> consisting of chemicals, metals, radiation, artificial food additives, sugar, and other modern toxins.

The excessive amounts of chemicals found in today's world effectively poison cells, which makes them sick, which then invites parasites to consume the toxic cells. Once their job of cleansing is done, the parasites spontaneously disappear. Parasites, like all microbes, spontaneously appear and disappear depending on the condition of one's internal environment. If you keep a clean internal environment, the clean up crew won't be called in. Internal hygiene is just as important as external hygiene.

There is a caveat to parasites. As parasites consume toxic matter from the body, they also produce excrement. Therefore, the more toxic you are the more parasites you will manifest, and the more parasite excrement will float around in your body. When this excrement is in small amounts, or when you have a healthy detox system, the excrement can be easily removed from your body. All is good in this instance.

Nature dictates that if you have excess toxicity you will attract excessive amounts of parasites. If additionally, you have a sluggish detox system the parasitic excrement could accumulate in your body and cause an infection. Typically, the parasites are blamed for causing the health problems but the truth is they manifested <u>after</u> your body was toxic, in order to remove the sick tissues caused by the toxins. Parasites simply just show up to cleanse a toxic body. Maintain a clean body that has a low toxic load, therefore parasites won't have a reason to manifest.

Remember, parasites are not found in clean organic grass-fed meat. There is no need to fear healthy meat. You can now relax and enjoy this healthful food.

Toxins Formed when Cooking Meat

Understand that when raw meat is cooked the proteins and fats are denatured and therefore are less utilizable in the body. Additionally, heat alteration produces toxins in the meat such as heterocyclic amines (HCA), advanced glycation end products (AGE), 4-hydroxynonenal (HNE), malondialdehyde (MDA), polycyclic aromatic hydrocarbons (PAH), glyoxal, and acrolein. These toxins have been proven to be carcinogenic. They are also known to cause inflammation, arthritis, Alzheimer's, Parkinson's, digestive issues, bloating, and other health disturbances.

Freezing Meat

I also recommend eating fresh meat and not frozen which is another form of denaturing the meat. Freezing the meat will kill the inherent probiotics in the meat, and decrease its ability to repopulate your gut microbiome.

Eating Fat with Your Meat

Raw meat, like all raw foods, helps to release toxins from the body. Because of this detoxification, it's important to eat raw fat with the raw meat. The raw fat binds to the released toxins and the toxins are later excreted. Additionally, the body assimilates protein and minerals more efficiently when raw fat is present. The body also absorbs the pigments in meat, myoglobin and hemoglobin, better when meat is eaten with fats. I like to eat my raw meat with little chunks of raw butter, avocado, sour cream, or simply drizzle olive oil on the meat.

There are many other reasons to eat raw meat, but I'll give you one more. If you want to build long lasting muscles that don't deflate after several days of not exercising, then raw meat is the answer. Since beef is muscle, it makes sense that eating muscle will also build muscle. Raw meat is also the easiest way to repair and rejuvenate cells. With all of the benefits of eating raw meat, you won't find me cooking the goodness out of it.

A Note about Meat, Chicken, and Fish

Yes, it's most beneficial to eat your meat raw. However, you may not feel like eating this way all of the time. I recommend that when you feel like eating cooked meat that you sear it, cook it below 212 degrees Fahrenheit, or use the sous vide method.

Twelve

FRESH ORGANIC PASTURE-RAISED RAW CHICKEN

I sometimes feel uneasy sharing about raw chicken because it's unconventional to many people. However, I've come to understand that raw chicken, just like the topic of microbes, has been misunderstood. If chickens are raised in the way that nature intended, in an organic and pasture-raised manner, they are safe and healthy to eat raw. Healthy chickens are meant to eat seeds, bugs, worms, larva, grasses, roots, and get ample sunlight and fresh air. Chicken is no different from eating raw fish or any other animal that's been raised cleanly, without chemicals, and humanely.

I like to eat chicken in the raw because it tastes delicious, and the unheated proteins and fats are recognized by my body, and therefore are easily utilizable. Conversely, when proteins and fats are heated their chemical, microbial, enzymatic, and energetic structures are altered and therefore cannot be incorporated into human tissues as easily. Raw chicken will rejuvenate and repair tissues that raw meat and raw fish cannot accomplish.

~ *I always feel noticeably good when I eat raw chicken.* ~

I always feel noticeably good when I eat raw chicken. It quickly soothes my nervous system. At a recent event I was eating raw chicken ceviche and four people gathered around me and tried it for the first time. They all exclaimed how delicious it was, and said they couldn't tell it was raw chicken. If you're worried about eating raw chicken please know that numerous people in my raw food community have eaten it for several decades and have never been sick.

One of my customers in Venice Beach, CA had been suffering from shaky hands for many years and asked me for my recommendation. I suggested that he eat some raw chicken, and sure enough after several weeks his shakes greatly reduced. This amazing recovery is possible because raw chicken is known to regenerate nerves. It is also good at healing various lung conditions, and is effective when eaten at the onset of a cold or flu. Raw chicken also promotes healthy skin and lymphatic system.

Raw chicken can be eaten as sashimi style or made into a ceviche. When made into a ceviche the chicken is "cold cooked" in fresh lemon juice. I soak the chicken in fresh lemon juice for 1-2 days in a glass jar, and allow the acidity of the lemon to "cold cook" the chicken. Using this method the chicken has a whitish "cooked" appearance and is softer and more nutritious than chicken that's been cooked with heat. The soft texture and lemony flavor is delightful to my senses.

I only source fresh organic pasture-raised chicken from a local butcher, organic market, or farm. I like to ask the butcher questions and find that they are usually happy to answer them. I make sure that the chickens were not fed soy or corn, even if the feed is organic. **I recommend eating only organic, pasture-raised chicken.**

Thirteen

FRESH ORGANIC GRASS-FED RAW LIVER

Traditional cultures are known to have thrived by eating organ meats, however this trend has disappeared in modern life. These traditional cultures instinctively knew that organ meats were more nutritious than other parts of the animal. Sometimes animals in the wild, when not too hungry, will only eat the abdominal organs. They instinctively know that organ meats are the preferred food for sustaining life. The healthiest organs to eat are raw liver, raw kidneys, raw heart, raw adrenals, and raw thyroid. However, the king of all organs is the liver because it's the most nutrient-dense.

A friend recently asked me why I would even consider eating raw liver. Well, the answer is quite simple: liver is the ultimate superfood! Raw liver contains more nutrients gram for gram than any other food. Raw liver contains an anti-fatigue factor which increases stamina in athletes. My athlete friends tell me that it gives them a great edge in their sport.

~ *Liver is the ultimate superfood!* ~

Raw liver is exceedingly high in all of the B vitamins, especially vitamin B12 which is only found in animal foods. However, the vitamin B12 in vegan foods is in a form that's unabsorbable in the body. A vitamin B12 deficiency can cause depression, paranoia, memory loss, anemia, intestinal problems, nerve issues, incontinence, and an inability to cope with stress. Liver is also high in vitamin B6, which helps to prevent infertility, neuropathy, depression, confusion, and seizures.

Raw liver is also high in minerals such as iron, zinc, selenium, sulfur, potassium, copper, magnesium, and chromium. It also contains high amounts of the fat-soluble vitamins A, D, E, and K2, and when grass-fed contains omega-3 fats. I used to have poor night vision, however since eating raw liver pate my eyesight has greatly improved. This improvement is due to the concentrated amounts of vitamin A.

As a former hairstylist, I worked with many toxic chemicals that imposed an excessive load on my liver. I use to notice dark circles under my eyes and a yellowish skin tone all over my body, which told me that I had an overloaded liver. In natural medicine it's generally accepted that like heals like, so when I started eating raw paleo foods I ate raw liver in order to detoxify and regenerate my own liver. The liver is an essential organ for the attainment of health because it performs approximately 2000 functions, therefore when it's functioning optimally overall health can improve.

My clients and I have seen many health improvements by eating raw liver, and you can too. However, make sure that the liver is **always organic and grass-fed** to ensure that it's free from toxins. Please see recipe section for ways to enjoy raw liver.

Fourteen

RAW FERMENTED FOODS

Hippocrates, the father of modern medicine, is known to have said that all disease begins in the gut. For the most part, this perspective still holds true in natural medicine today. It's well known that a <u>deficiency</u> or <u>imbalance</u> of gut microorganisms will result in systemic health problems. Natasha McBride, MD, expert on gut health, states that an imbalance in the digestive system will adversely affect the brain. [20] To improve gut health the resident strains of bacteria must first be reintroduced into the gut microbiome. An easy way to restore your microbiome is to regularly eat various types of fermented foods, and most importantly a wide variety of raw omnivorous foods. Each type of raw food contains probiotics that will in turn feed the numerous species of bacteria in your gut.

Due to the many probiotic bacteria found in fermented foods, I suggest eating them on a daily basis. There are ten times more bacteria in the human body than there are cells. In a way, people are a cluster of walking bacteria.

A healthy person with a balanced microbiome has about six pounds of beneficial bacteria in their gut. Humans are very dependent on these wonderful bacteria.

My friend Hanna, who's known as The Kombucha Momma, likes to tell people that she's "bacteria powered." She claims that she gets a lot of energy from the good bacteria in fermented foods. Due to the synergistic nature between humans and bacteria, she coined a new word claiming that humans are bacteria sapiens. I fully concur.

Beneficial bacteria have several roles in the body such as chelating heavy metals and pesticides, helping the body to manufacture B vitamins, and improving digestion. They even cleanse dangerous waste from the body! You will be pleased by introducing the new taste of fermented foods, along with their wide-reaching health benefits.

Another function of bacteria is to keep the immune system healthy. Did you know that 75 percent of our immune system resides in our gut in the form of bacteria? These gut bacteria also prevent pathogenic bacteria from overpopulating, and therefore are your allies in preventing infections.

I consume a wide array of fermented foods such as Jun, raw dairy kefir, raw dairy yogurt, kvass, coconut water kefir, raw kimchi, raw sauerkraut, and homemade lacto-fermented pickles. I like to have these foods as a side dish with my meals. The bacteria in these foods predigest the hard-to-break-down components of the food, thus making it easier to absorb the food's nutrients. You can also drink the juice (brine) of fermented veggies for even greater digestive benefits. The brine is especially good for constipation and an upset stomach.

~ *Raw milk is amazing, but when transformed into*
cultured milk it becomes magical. ~

I'm excited to tell you about one of my favorite fermented foods, a home-made raw dairy kefir that's similar to cultured milk. In Persia it's believed that an angel showed Abraham how to prepare a yogurt-like drink that gave him fertility and longevity. Persian women believe that cultured milk products are responsible for their notoriously healthy skin. In Turkish, kefir means "feel good," and true to this old legend I feel deeply happy soon after having my homemade kefir. Raw milk is amazing, but when transformed into cultured milk it becomes magical. During this culturing process calcium, phosphorus, and many other nutrients become much more bioavailable to your body.

The culturing of raw fermented kefir produces lactic acid which acts as a digestive antiseptic, aiding in the health of the intestinal tract. The benefits are so great that in 1959 they called acidophilus "nature's gastro-intestinal antibiotic." Next time you are experiencing diarrhea, constipation, or any intestinal discomfort you can consider having some raw dairy kefir; nature's antibiotic.

You can make your own kefir at home by using kefir grains and raw whole milk. When you make raw kefir at home you know exactly where everything is sourced from, and there are no thickeners, preservatives, sugars, or suspicious natural flavors. Beware that all of the dairy kefir you buy in commercial grocery stores has been pasteurized. This means that many of its nutrients have been altered or destroyed. The result is a dead product that may contain some beneficial bacteria. However, the bacteria are not that useful anymore because the kefir has lost its nutritional synergy. It makes much more sense to leave nature alone, because nature always knows best.

> ~ *It makes sense to leave nature alone, because*
> *nature always knows best.* ~

Note: It's been believed for many decades that in order to restore gut bacteria you can simply take a probiotic pill. However, since these pills contain only 5-15 species of bacteria they are unable to feed all 1,000 species of resident bacteria in the gut. The practice of taking probiotic pills will overfeed several species while ignoring the other 990 odd resident species. This will result in an imbalance of gut bacteria in the long term, which could compound your heath issues. It's well known that a deficiency of gut bacteria can cause disease, however an imbalance of gut bacteria can also cause disease. I therefore recommend you eat as many different kinds of raw fermented foods and a wide variety of raw omnivorous foods so that you'll feed all 1,000 species of bacteria in the gut.

Fifteen

FRESH ORGANIC RAW GREEN JUICE

Green juice is essential on the raw paleo diet because it performs many needed functions. When I drink green juice it feels as if I'm taking in pure life. It feels refreshingly good as it hydrates, cleanses, and nourishes my whole body. This great feeling occurs because fresh vegetable juice contains highly bioavailable water, minerals, vitamins, enzymes, chlorophyll, life force, and many wonderful phytonutrients. Green juice is an important part of the raw paleo diet and must be drunk daily.

~ *Green juice is an important part of the raw paleo diet*
and must be drunk daily. ~

Green juice is something I especially turn to whenever I feel that something is not quite right in my body. When I'm feeling this way I drink more than my usual amount of one pint, and the problem usually resolves itself. Green juice keeps my body in the correct pH balance, improves my bowel movements, keeps my skin glowing, enhances my digestion, and gives me energy.

Nature's brilliance is such that green juice will alkalize your body without alkalizing the acidic parts of your digestive tract. This is unlike the man-made alkaline water that's become popular nowadays which can alkalize your stomach and cause indigestion. To properly digest protein foods we need to have the correct pH balance in our entire digestive tract. If you're drinking 8-16oz of green juice daily you should have an optimal pH balance.

The green juice that I'm referring to is homemade, fresh, and unpasteurized. I've found a way to make juicing a lot easier by making a half gallon (64oz) of green juice at time, which lasts me for 3 days.

Note: When you buy drinks such as vegetable juice, coconut water, and fruit juice, you must look for unpasteurized, raw, and non-high pressure processing (HPP) products. HPP products are not truly raw.

My Favorite Green Juice Recipe:
60% organic celery
30% organic cucumber
5-10% organic parsley
5% organic cilantro (only add after several months of juicing)

Parsley is known to remove heavy metals from the cells. Some people like to further increase this effect by adding cilantro to their juice. However, be very careful because even though these two herbs pull heavy metals out the cells, they do not get the heavy metals out of the body. Removing too many toxins out of your cells, too fast, can congest and overwhelm your detox system which will cause unnecessary health problems. To reduce the chance of such problems start out by using only parsley, and after a few months you can add cilantro. You could also add raw cow cream, raw egg, or olive oil to your juice which will help to bind toxins and increase the absorption of the antioxidants (pigments) in the juice. Adding bentonite clay to your juice will also help to bind the toxins that have been released from your cells.

You can get creative with your vegetable juice by adding different vegetables such as beets, carrots, cabbage, broccoli, spinach, kale, or zucchini. The greater variety of vegetables that you include, the wider array of nutrients you will receive. Enjoy the fun and beauty of mixing the various colors together. It's essential to drink fresh green juice every day.

How to make your Green Juice last for 3 days:
- Once your juice is made, pour it into 8 or 12oz glass jars.
- Add 1/2 teaspoon of raw honey in each jar as a preservative.
- Fill the glass jars all the way to the very top, leaving no air in them.
- Seal jar tightly.
- Place in refrigerator.

Three Types of Juicers:
The vegetable juicers that I recommend are the Green Star twin gear, Omega J8006 single auger, and the Breville Juice Fountain Plus centrifugal juicer.

My favorite juicer is the Green Star, using a wooden push stick rather than a plastic one. A plastic push stick can scrape against the metal gears causing pieces of plastic to end up in the juice.

Whichever juicer you choose make sure that it contains mostly stainless steel parts, rather than plastic. Plastic parts contain dioxin and other petrochemicals that could be released into your juice.

Sixteen

MY DAILY MEAL PLAN

I suggest you transition into this new way of eating at a pace that's suitable for you. I found that after consistently eating nutrient-dense foods I am now nutritionally satisfied and no longer have the old cravings. I personally eat 80% raw foods, the rest cooked.

~ *No matter what you eat, enjoy it and give thanks.* ~

Nowadays I eat the basic raw paleo foods, but when you're first starting out you may want to dress your meals with ingredients that make it fun and enjoyable. I've also made a lifestyle change that whenever I leave home for the day I pack a medium-size cooler with my glass mason jars filled with raw foods. Have fun on this new journey!

This eating program outlines what works for me, however please listen to your own body and use discernment to know what works for you.

Raw Paleo

<u>Breakfast</u>: 7-9 AM
I like to choose from one of the following:

- 12oz glass fresh organic green juice
- 8oz organic raw dairy kefir (cow or goat)
- 1 piece organic raw butter banana cream pie (see recipe in raw butter recipes)
- 2 slices of organic raw cheese with raw honey
- 2 pasture-raised raw eggs eaten Rocky style
- Raw smoothie with 8oz organic raw milk and fresh seasonal fruit (see smoothie chapter)

<u>Lunch</u>: 11-1 PM
I like to choose from one of the following:

- Organic avocado, a few squares of organic raw cheese, and kimchi drizzled with olive oil
- 8oz grass-fed raw meat dish
- Organic raw milk smoothie (see smoothie chapter)
- A mono meal of seasonal organic fruit (a mono meal is when you eat only one type of fruit until you're fully satiated)

<u>Snack</u>: 3-4 PM
I like to choose from one of the following:

- A fruit meal with a raw fat such as strawberries and raw cream
- 12oz fresh organic green juice
- 1 organic avocado
- Fermented veggies

<u>Dinner</u>: 6-7 PM
I like to choose from one of the following:

- 1 cup of grass-fed raw meat (bison tartare, beef tartare, chicken ceviche, or fish ceviche) eaten with a raw fat (sour cream, raw butter, avocado, olive oil)
- Organic raw dairy kefir smoothie
- 1 piece of organic raw butter banana cream pie
- Organic leafy greens salad with vegetables, and olive oil-fresh lemon juice dressing
- 1 cup bone broth with avocado and fermented veggies

<u>A Note for Men</u>: If you want to increase muscle mass I recommend eating raw red meat after your workout. Raw eggs, raw meat, and raw milk are great muscle building foods.

Seventeen

Know Your Food Source

Please read over this section before making any of these delicious recipes.

It's important to ask questions about your food, such as where it came from, methods of growing, and other such questions.

A great place to source your food is from local organic farmers markets, local co-ops, or specialty butcher shops. You can also contact your local Weston A. Price chapter leader for a food resource guide.

Questions to Ask at the Farmers Market

Raising of Animals:
- Is the animal raised on organic feed?
- If the feed is not organic, ask if it is GMO free?
- Are the animals out on green pasture 24/7, or only a part of the day?
- Are the animals grass-fed and grass finished?

<u>Raising Bees:</u>
- What kind of plants do the bees pollinate?
- Are the bees fed sugar water during the winter?
- Are the bees ever given antibiotics?
- Are your bees transported in order to pollinate commercial crops? (this inhumane practice is destructive to the bees).

<u>Growing of Produce</u>:
- Is the farm in an isolated area, or near a freeway where there is increased contamination?
- What kind of water is used: chlorinated, fluoridated, spring, or well?
- Are artificial fertilizers used? (natural fertilizers come from animal manure, bird droppings, or fish emulsion)
- Are any artificial chemicals of <u>any</u> kind ever used?
- Are waxes used on the produce? (most waxes are petroleum based)

How to Buy the Healthiest Products

<u>Raw Honey</u>:
- Raw (must <u>also</u> include one of these descriptions: unheated, unpasteurized, uncooked, or cold packed).

<u>Raw Coconut Oil</u>:
- Organic.
- Raw and cold pressed (label must say both raw <u>and</u> cold pressed).
- Unrefined.

<u>Raw Eggs</u>:
- Organic.
- Pasture-raised (<u>free range</u> and <u>cage free</u> are not pasture-raised).

- Preferably Fertile.
- Corn-free and soy-free.
- Non-irradiated/pasteurized.

Raw Dairy:
- Organic.
- Grass-fed.
- Unpasteurized
- Non-homogenized.
**You can find local raw dairy sources at www.realmilk.com.

Red Meat:
- Organic.
- Grass-fed <u>and</u> grass-finished.
- Fresh and never frozen.

Chicken:
- Organic.
- Pasture-raised.
- Corn-free and soy-free.
- Fresh and never frozen.

Fish:
- Wild-caught (farmed fish is toxic for people and planet).
- Preferably never frozen.
- Not from the Gulf of Mexico (after the oil spill of 2010 some large health food store chains do not say which part of USA their fish comes from).

Fruit and Vegetables:
- Preferably biodynamic.
- Organic or sustainably-raised are fine.

- Locally grown (ideally grow your own).
- Seasonal.
- Preferably never frozen.
- Non-irradiated (conventional produce is oftentimes irradiated).

Dried Herbs and Spices:
- Organic.
- Non-irradiated.

Our current food system is unreliable and is not intended for the health of people or planet. When you buy from an organic local farmer you are investing in food that will support you, the farmer, and the planet. Buying from a farmers market allows you to build community, and connects you to your food.

The Raw Paleo Recipes

Kitchen Equipment Required:
Vitamix blender
Food processor
Sharp knifes
Spatula
Bamboo cutting board
Potato peeler (to peel cucumbers if they have been waxed)
Micro-plane (a fine grater)
Nut milk bag (a fine mesh bag for squeezing the lemon out of the chicken)
Small stainless tea strainer (for squeezing the juice out of the grated ginger)
Glass measuring cups
Measuring spoons

Recipe Notes:

1. After preparing the recipes I place the food in glass jars and store in the refrigerator.
2. When you're making the raw butter recipes (Mango Butter Pudding or Bone Marrow Mousse), if they get chunky or gritty just continue blending until a creamy consistency is achieved.
3. For most of the recipes I call for "softened" butter. Simply place the raw butter on a counter for several hours at room temperature until it softens.

Eighteen

RAW CONDIMENTS

1) <u>Raw Mayonnaise</u>

<u>Ingredients</u>:
- 2 organic pasture-raised raw egg yolks
- 1 tablespoon fresh squeezed lemon juice
- 1 teaspoon organic raw apple cider vinegar
- 1 cup organic cold pressed olive oil
- 1 teaspoon raw mustard
- 1 teaspoon raw honey
- ¼ teaspoon Himalayan salt

<u>Instructions</u>:
Add egg yolk, lemon juice, apple cider vinegar, olive oil, raw mustard, and raw honey into a wide mouth glass jar and use an immersion blender to blend. Start by pulsing the blender, and blend for 2 minutes. Serve and eat immediately, or place in a glass jar and store in the refrigerator. Shelf life is 1 month.

2) <u>Raw Mustard</u>

<u>Ingredients</u>:
3 tablespoons yellow mustard seeds
3 tablespoons brown mustard seeds
3 ounces of sparkling mineral water
2 tablespoons organic raw apple cider vinegar
1 tablespoon raw honey

<u>Instructions</u>:
Add the mustard seeds and apple cider vinegar to a one pint glass jar, fill with sparkling water, and seal the jar. Let the jar sit at room temperature for 24 hours. Add the mixture from the jar into a Vitamix blender, add honey, and blend until it reaches a smooth consistency. Serve and eat immediately, or place in a glass jar and store in the refrigerator. Shelf life is 6 months.

3) <u>Raw Pickles</u>

<u>Step 1</u>: **Cutting the Cucumbers**
<u>Ingredients</u>:
- 2 peeled organic cucumbers

<u>Instructions</u>:
Slice the cucumbers lengthwise, long enough to fit into a 32oz quart jar. Cut off and discard the soft-seed core section.

<u>Step 2</u>: **Pickle Brine**
<u>Ingredients</u>:
- 1 cup organic raw apple cider vinegar
- 1 cup sparkling mineral water
- 1 tablespoon raw honey

Instructions:
Add apple cider vinegar, sparkling mineral water, and honey into a Vitamix blender and blend until well mixed. Place the sliced cucumbers into a wide-mouth glass quart jar. Add blended pickle brine into the jar until it completely covers the cucumbers. Seal and place the jar in the refrigerator for 3-4 days. Serve and eat immediately, or place in a glass jar and store in the refrigerator. Shelf life is 5 days.

4) <u>Raw Coconut Cream Recipe</u>

Ingredients:
- 4 mature organic coconuts (dark brown)

Instructions:
Look for coconuts that do not have mold anywhere on them, especially on the two eyes and one mouth. Dark spots anywhere on the coconut are also not a good sign. If the eyes or mouth is elevated, do not buy the coconut. This means that the water is fermenting, and could possibly have moldy coconut meat inside.

The two eyes are hard but the mouth is soft. Therefore, poke a hole into the soft mouth, and drain the coconut water into a 32oz glass jar.

Put on a pair of heavy duty gloves and crack the coconut open with a hammer. This is done by hammering around the equator of the coconut until it cracks open.

Shuck out the coconut meat using an oyster shucker. Add the coconut meat into a food processor and blend into fine chunks. Place the coconut pieces onto a tray in a dehydrator. Warm the coconut pieces in the dehydrator at 100 degrees Fahrenheit, for approximately 30 minutes.

Put the warm coconut pieces through a Green Star juicer or Champion juicer to make the cream. Serve and eat immediately, or place in a glass jar and store in the refrigerator. Shelf life is 5 days.

Note: Coconut cream is still edible after being in the refrigerator for many months. It simply becomes richer in probiotics the longer it stays in the refrigerator. However, in this state it's only palatable when used in smoothies.

If the coconut cream comes out of the juicer lumpy, gritty, or too solid it means that your shreds are not warm enough. To ensure that your coconut pieces are warm enough, you can use a space heater to heat the room.

Nineteen

RAW BUTTER RECIPES
(eat anytime, even as a meal)

1) <u>**Raw Mango Butter Pudding**</u>

<u>Ingredients</u>:
- 1 ripe organic mango (peeled and cut up into small pieces for blender)
- ½ cup organic grass-fed raw butter (softened)
- 2 organic pasture-raised raw eggs
- Fresh squeezed juice of 1 organic lime or lemon
- 1-2 tablespoons raw honey

<u>Instructions</u>:
Add the mango, butter, eggs, lemon, and honey into a Vitamix blender and blend until it reaches a smooth consistency. Serve and eat immediately, or place in a glass jar and store in the refrigerator. Shelf life is 5 days.

2) <u>Raw Creamy Papaya Custard</u>

<u>Ingredients</u>:
- 1 whole organic papaya (peel and remove the seeds)
- 4 tablespoons organic grass-fed raw butter (softened)
- 2 organic pasture-raised raw eggs
- 1-2 tablespoons raw honey

<u>Instructions</u>:
Add the papaya, butter, eggs, and honey into a Vitamix blender and blend until it reaches a smooth consistency. Serve and eat immediately, or place in a glass jar and store in the refrigerator. Shelf life is 5 days.

3) <u>Raw Chocolate Mousse</u>

<u>Ingredients</u>:
- ½ pound organic grass-fed raw butter (softened)
- 4 organic pasture-raised raw eggs
- ½ cup raw cacao powder (add more if you love chocolate)
- 3 tablespoons raw honey

<u>Instructions</u>:
Add the butter, eggs, cacao powder, and honey into a Vitamix blender and blend until it reaches a smooth consistency. Add 1-2 more eggs if you want a creamier mousse. If you want to make fudge instead of mousse, then only use 2 eggs in the entire recipe. Serve and eat immediately, or place in a glass jar and store in the refrigerator. Shelf life is 2 weeks.

4) <u>Raw Mint Chocolate Mousse</u>

<u>Ingredients</u>:
- ½ pound organic grass-fed raw butter (softened)
- 4 organic pasture-raised raw eggs
- ½ cup raw cacao powder
- 3 tablespoons raw honey
- 1-2 teaspoons organic peppermint extract

<u>Instructions</u>:
Add the butter, eggs, cacao powder, honey, and peppermint extract into a Vitamix blender and blend until it reaches a smooth consistency. Serve and eat immediately, or place in a glass jar and store in the refrigerator. Shelf life is 2 weeks.

5) <u>Raw Banana Cream Butter Pie</u>

<u>Step1</u>: **Crust**
<u>Ingredients</u>:
- ¾ cup presoaked raw walnuts
- ¾ cup presoaked unpasteurized raw almonds (most almonds have been pasteurized)
- 2 tablespoons organic grass-fed raw butter (softened)
- 1 tablespoon raw honey
- 3 tablespoons raw cacao powder (optional)

<u>Instructions</u>:
Use a food processor (not a blender) to mix the walnuts, almonds, butter, and honey until it reaches a smooth consistency. Press the

mixture into an 8 inch round Springform pie pan with your hands to make the crust.

Step 2: **Filling**
Ingredients:
- 4 ripe organic bananas (1-2 brown spots on them)
- Remainder of the 1 pound softened raw butter
- 3 organic pasture-raised raw eggs
- 5 pitted organic medjool dates
- 1 teaspoon raw vanilla bean powder
- Fresh squeezed juice of ½ an organic lemon
- 2 tablespoons raw honey

Instructions:
Add the bananas, butter, eggs, pitted dates, vanilla bean powder, lemon juice, and honey into a Vitamix blender and blend until it reaches a smooth consistency. Pour the mixture onto the crust and put in the refrigerator to set for 6-8 hours. For a faster setting time put in the freezer for two hours.

Step 3: **Frosting**
Ingredients:
- 12oz organic grass-fed raw cream
- 1 tablespoon raw honey

Instructions:
Place cream and honey into a glass bowl and mix with a hand mixer. Be careful not to over mix the cream or you'll have butter! When the cream thickens into a frosting, use a spatula and frost the pie. Serve and eat immediately, or place in glass jars and store in the refrigerator. Shelf life is 5 days.

6) Raw Butter Cream

Ingredients:
- ¾ pound organic grass-fed raw butter (softened)
- 3 organic pasture-raised raw eggs
- ½ teaspoon raw vanilla bean powder
- 2 tablespoons raw honey

Instructions:
Add butter, eggs, vanilla bean powder, and honey into a Vitamix blender and blend until it reaches a smooth consistency. Serve and eat immediately, or place in a glass jar and store in the refrigerator. Shelf life is 5 days.

Note:
The above recipe can also be used as an alternative frosting on the raw banana cream butter pie.

7) Raw Pineapple Butter Blast

Ingredients:
- 1½ cups organic pineapple cut into small chunks
- 2 tablespoons organic grass-fed raw butter (softened)
- 2 organic pasture-raised raw eggs
- ½ organic avocado
- 1 teaspoon raw vanilla bean powder
- 1 tablespoon raw honey

Instructions:
Add the pineapple, butter, eggs, avocado, vanilla bean powder, and honey into a Vitamix blender and blend until a reaches a smooth consistency.

Serve and eat immediately, or place in a glass jar and store in the refrigerator. Shelf life is 5 days.

8) <u>Raw Persimmon Smoothie</u>

<u>Ingredients</u>:
- 2 super ripe soft organic Hachiya persimmons
- 2 tablespoons organic grass-fed raw butter (softened)
- 1-2 organic pasture-raised raw eggs
- 1 cup fresh organic raw coconut water
- 1 tablespoons raw honey

<u>Instructions</u>:
Add the persimmons, butter, eggs, coconut water, and honey into a Vitamix blender and blend until it reaches a smooth consistency. Serve and eat immediately, or place in a glass jar and store in the refrigerator. Shelf life is 5 days.

9) <u>Raw Peanut Butter Squares</u>

<u>Ingredients</u>:
- 1/3 pound organic grass-fed raw butter (softened)
- 1 cup raw wild jungle peanut butter (found at local Co-ops)
- ½ cup raw honey

<u>Instructions</u>:
Mix the butter, peanut butter, and honey together with a hand mixer or food processor. Place the mixture into a glass Pyrex dish and pat down evenly with your hands until it's flat. Chill in the refrigerator for 4-6 hours. Take dish out of the refrigerator and cut into squares. Serve and

eat immediately, or place in glass jars and store in the refrigerator. Shelf life is 2 weeks.

10) <u>Raw Raspberry Butter</u>

<u>Ingredients</u>:
- 1 cup fresh organic raspberries
- ½ cup organic grass-fed raw butter (softened)
- 1 tablespoon raw honey

<u>Instructions</u>:
Add raspberries, butter, and honey into a Vitamix blender and blend until it reaches a smooth consistency. Place the mixture into a glass Pyrex dish and pat down evenly with your hands until it's flat. Chill in the refrigerator for 4-6 hours. Take dish out of the refrigerator and cut into fun shapes with a cookie cutter. Serve and eat immediately, or place in glass jars and store in the refrigerator. Shelf life is 2 weeks.

11) <u>Raw Butter Tartine</u>

<u>Ingredients</u>:
- 2 slices lightly toasted organic sour dough bread
- 4 tablespoons organic grass-fed raw butter (softened)
- ½ teaspoon organic cinnamon powder
- 1 tablespoon raw honey

<u>Instructions</u>:
Spread the softened butter on the toast, drizzle with honey, and sprinkle with cinnamon. This is a great party treat. Serve and eat immediately.

12) <u>Raw Carob Butter Pudding</u>

<u>Ingredients</u>:
- ½ pound organic grass-fed raw butter (softened)
- 2 organic pasture-raised raw eggs
- 2 ripe organic bananas
- 4 tablespoons raw carob powder
- 1 teaspoon raw vanilla bean powder
- 2 tablespoons raw honey

<u>Instructions</u>:
Add butter, eggs, bananas, carob powder, vanilla bean powder, and honey into a Vitamix blender and blend until it reaches a smooth consistency. Serve and eat immediately, or place in a glass jar and store in the refrigerator. Shelf life is 5 days.

13) <u>Raw Garlic Honey Butter</u>

<u>Ingredients</u>:
- 4 tablespoons organic grass-fed raw butter
- 2 fresh organic garlic cloves (micro-planed or pressed)
- 1 teaspoon raw honey

<u>Instructions</u>:
Place the butter in a glass jar with a tightly closed lid. Lightly melt the butter in bowl of warm water. Open the jar, add garlic and honey. Shake well. Serve and eat immediately, or store in the refrigerator. Shelf life is 2 weeks.

14) <u>Raw Chocolate Almond Fudge Swirl</u>

<u>Ingredients</u>:
- ½ pound organic grass-fed raw butter (softened)
- 4 tablespoons organic raw almond butter
- 2 organic pasture-raised raw eggs
- 4 pitted organic medjool dates
- 1 ripe organic banana
- 4 tablespoons raw cacao powder
- 1 teaspoon raw vanilla bean powder
- 1 tablespoons raw honey

<u>Instructions</u>:
<u>Step 1</u>: **Base**
Add butter, almond butter, eggs, dates, banana, vanilla bean powder, and honey <u>(except cacao powder)</u> into a Vitamix blender and blend until it reaches a smooth consistency. Pour half of the mixture into a glass Pyrex pan.

<u>Step 2</u>: **Chocolate Mix**
Add 4 tablespoons of cacao powder into the rest of the mixture that's still in the Vitamix blender and blend again.

<u>Step 3</u>: **Swirling**
Pour the blended cacao mixture over the first mixture that's in the Pyrex pan, swirling it in using a wooden spoon. Place in the refrigerator for 4-6 hours until it sets. Cut the hardened fudge into bar size shapes. Serve and eat immediately, or place in a glass jar and store in the refrigerator. Shelf life is 2 weeks.

15) <u>Warm Butter Drink</u>

<u>Ingredients</u>:
- 1 cup warm filtered water
- 2 tablespoons organic grass-fed raw butter
- 1 teaspoon raw honey

<u>Instructions</u>:
Warm a small pot of water on the stove to just under boiling. Add butter and honey to warm water, stir, and drink. This recipe is great for digestion.

16) <u>Raw Chai Butter Pudding</u>

<u>Ingredients</u>:
- ½ pound organic grass-fed raw butter (softened)
- ¼ cup organic grass-fed raw milk
- 3 organic pasture-raised raw eggs
- 1 teaspoon raw vanilla bean powder
- ½ teaspoon organic cardamom powder
- ½ teaspoon organic ginger powder
- ¼ teaspoon organic clove powder
- 2 shakes organic cinnamon powder
- 2 tablespoons raw honey

<u>Instructions</u>:
Add butter, milk, eggs, vanilla bean powder, cardamom powder, ginger powder, clove powder, cinnamon powder, and honey into a Vitamix blender and blend until it reaches a smooth consistency. Serve and eat immediately, or place in a glass jar and store in the refrigerator. Shelf life is 7 days.

17) Refreshing Raw Grapefruit Butter Snack

Ingredients:
- ½ pound organic grass-fed raw butter (softened)
- 3 organic pasture-raised raw eggs
- ½ cup fresh squeezed organic grapefruit juice
- 2 tablespoons raw honey

Instructions:
Add butter, eggs, grapefruit juice, and honey into a Vitamix blender and blend until it reaches a smooth consistency. Serve and eat immediately, or place in a glass jar and store in the refrigerator. Shelf life is 7 days.

18) Raw Dark Chocolate Spirulina Pudding

Ingredients:
- 1 ripe organic avocado
- 10 pitted organic medjool dates
- 3 tablespoons organic grass-fed raw butter (softened)
- 4 tablespoons raw cacao powder
- ½ teaspoon raw vanilla bean powder
- ¼ teaspoon Hawaiian spirulina powder
- 5 tablespoons filtered water

Instructions:
Add the avocado, pitted dates, butter, cacao powder, vanilla bean powder, spirulina powder, and water into a Vitamix blender and blend until it reaches a smooth consistency. Serve and eat immediately, or place in a glass jar and store in the refrigerator. Shelf life is 7 days.

19) <u>Raw Pineapple Cheesecake</u>

<u>Step 1</u>: **Crust**
<u>Ingredients</u>:
- 2 cups presoaked unpasteurized raw almonds (most almonds have been pasteurized)
- 2 tablespoons organic grass-fed raw butter (softened)
- 1 tablespoon raw honey

<u>Instructions</u>:
Add almonds, butter, and honey to a food processor and mix until it reaches a smooth consistency, or leave slightly chunky if desired. Press the mixture into an 8 inch round Springform pie pan with your hands to make the crust.

<u>Step 2</u>: **Pie filling**
<u>Ingredients</u>:
- 8oz organic grass-fed raw cream cheese (allow to soften on a counter for a few hours prior to use)
- ½ cup organic grass-fed raw cream (old cream that has soured is also fine)
- ½ pound organic grass-fed raw butter (softened)
- 2 organic pasture-raised raw eggs
- 1 cup chopped organic pineapple
- 4 pitted organic medjool dates
- 2 tablespoons raw honey

<u>Instructions</u>:
Add pineapple, cream, butter, eggs, pitted dates, and honey into a Vitamix blender and blend until it reaches a smooth consistency. Pour

the mixture onto the crust. Using a wooden spoon add the softened cream cheese a few inches apart into the pineapple mixture, and swirl together. Allow it to set in the refrigerator for 4-6 hours. Serve and eat immediately, or place in glass jars and store in the refrigerator. Shelf life is 7 days.

20) <u>Raw Pumpkin Seed Butter</u>

<u>Ingredients</u>:
- 2 cups presoaked raw pumpkin seeds
- 4 tablespoons organic grass-fed raw butter (softened)
- 2 organic pasture-raised raw eggs
- 1 tablespoon organic raw coconut oil
- 2 tablespoons raw honey

<u>Instructions</u>:
Add the pumpkin seeds, eggs, butter, coconut oil, and honey into a Vitamix blender and blend until it reaches a smooth consistency. Serve and eat immediately, or place in a glass jar and store in the refrigerator. Shelf life is 2 weeks.

21) <u>Raw Decadent Blackberry Cheesecake</u>

<u>Step1</u>: **Blackberry Sauce**
<u>Ingredients</u>:
- ½ cup fresh organic blackberries
- Fresh squeezed juice of 1 organic lemon
- 1 teaspoon raw honey

Instructions:
Add the blackberries, lemon juice, and raw honey into a Vitamix blender and blend until it reaches a smooth consistency.

Step 2: **Cheesecake**
Ingredients:
- 6 tablespoons organic grass-fed raw cheese (allow to soften on a counter for a few hours prior to use)
- 5 pitted organic medjool dates
- 1 organic pasture-raised raw egg
- ¼ teaspoon raw vanilla bean powder
- 1 tablespoon raw honey

Instructions:
Add the cheese, dates, egg, vanilla bean powder, and honey into a Vitamix blender and blend until it reaches a smooth consistency. Place into a circular mold or round bowl and put in the refrigerator for 4-6 hours until it sets. Serve and eat immediately, or place in a glass jar and store in the refrigerator. Shelf life is 7 days.

Step 3: **Drizzle Sauce**
Instructions:
Drizzle blackberry sauce on top of the cheesecake.

Twenty

RAW DAIRY SHAKES
(your daily delights)

1) <u>Raw Spicy Goat Milkshake</u>

<u>Ingredients</u>:
- 1½ cups organic grass-fed raw goat milk
- 2 organic pasture-raised raw eggs
- 2 shakes organic cinnamon powder
- 2 shakes organic nutmeg powder
- 2 shakes organic clove powder
- 3 shakes organic cayenne pepper
- 2 tablespoons raw honey

<u>Instructions</u>:
Add goat milk, eggs, cinnamon, nutmeg, clove, cayenne pepper, and honey into a Vitamix blender and blend until it reaches a smooth consistency. Serve and eat immediately, or place in a glass jar and store in the refrigerator. Shelf life is 7 days.

2) <u>Raw Pineapple Digestive Smoothie</u>

<u>Ingredients</u>:
- 1½ cups chopped organic pineapple
- 1 cup organic grass-fed raw yogurt or raw dairy kefir
- ¼ cup grass-fed raw butter (softened)
- 1 organic pasture-raised raw egg
- ¼ teaspoon raw vanilla bean powder
- 2 tablespoons raw honey

<u>Instructions</u>:
Add pineapple, yogurt, butter, egg, vanilla bean powder, and honey into a Vitamix blender and blend until it reaches a smooth consistency. Serve and eat immediately, or place in a glass jar and store in the refrigerator. Shelf life is 7 days.

3) <u>Raw Beautiful Skin Smoothie</u>

<u>Ingredients</u>:
- 1 peeled and chopped organic cucumber
- 6 peeled organic kiwis
- 1 ripe organic avocado
- 1 handful fresh organic mint
- Fresh juice of 2 organic limes
- ¼ cup organic grass-fed raw cream
- 1-2 tablespoons raw honey

<u>Instructions</u>:
Add cucumber, kiwis, avocado, fresh mint, lime juice, cream, and honey into a Vitamix blender and blend until it reaches a smooth consistency.

Serve and eat immediately, or place in a glass jar and store in the refrigerator. Shelf life is 5 days.

4) Raw Golden Milk

Ingredients:
- 1½ cups organic grass-fed raw milk
- 3 tablespoons fresh organic turmeric root juice
- 1 tablespoon raw honey

Instructions:
Step 1: **Turmeric Juice**
Juice the turmeric root in a home juicer, or grate it on a zester, and squeeze it through a metal tea strainer.

Step 2: **Milkshake**
Add milk, turmeric juice, and honey into a glass mason jar, seal tightly and shake well. You can also add ingredients into a Vitamix blender and blend until it reaches a smooth consistency. Serve and eat immediately, or place in a glass jar and store in the refrigerator. Shelf life is 5 days.

5) Raw Kefir Energy Shake

Ingredients:
- 1½ cups organic grass-fed raw dairy kefir (goat or cow)
- 3 tablespoons raw cacao powder
- 1 tablespoon raw coconut oil
- 2 tablespoons raw honey
- ½ cup soaked and dehydrated pecans

Instructions:

Step 1: **Milkshake**

Blend dairy kefir, cacao powder, coconut oil, and honey into Vitamix blender and blend until it reaches a smooth consistency.

Step 2: **Pecans**

Add pecans and blend quickly on the pulse setting. Allow pecans to remain somewhat chunky. Serve and eat immediately, or place in a glass jar and store in the refrigerator. Shelf life is 7 days.

6) **Raw Coconut Cleansing Cocktail**

Ingredients:
- 1 cup fresh organic raw coconut cream (see coconut cream recipe page 59)
- 1 organic pasture-raised raw egg
- Fresh juice of 3 organic limes
- Fresh juice ½ organic grapefruit
- 2 tablespoons raw honey

Instructions:

Add coconut cream, egg, lime juice, grapefruit juice, and honey into a Vitamix blender and blend until it reaches a smooth consistency. Serve and eat immediately, or place in a glass jar and store in the refrigerator. Shelf life is 5 days.

7) **Raw Egg Cocktail**

Ingredients:
- 1 organic pasture-raised raw egg
- 2 tablespoons organic raw coconut oil (soften in a bowl of warm water)
- 1 tablespoon raw honey

Instructions:

Melt the coconut oil by placing the jar in hot water. Add the egg, co-conut oil, and honey into a Vitamix blender or hand mixer and shoot it Rocky Style! Drink this immediately, because it will harden in cold temperatures.

8) **Raw Bedtime Shake**

Ingredients:
- 2 cups organic grass-fed raw milk
- 1 organic pasture-raised raw egg
- 2 tablespoons organic ginger juice
- 1-2 tablespoons raw honey

Instructions:

Step 1: **Ginger Juice**

Juice the ginger in a home juicer, or grate on a microplane or cheese grater. Squeeze through a metal tea strainer.

Step 2: **Milkshake**

Fill a 1 pint glass mason jar 3/4 of the way with milk. Add egg, ginger juice, and honey and close the lid tightly. Shake mason jar vigorously until all ingredients are mixed. Serve and eat immediately, or place in a glass jar and store in the refrigerator. Shelf life is 5 days.

9) **Raw Coconut Glowing Skin Tonic**

Ingredients:
- 1 cup freshly made organic raw coconut cream (or raw dairy cream)
- 1 cup chopped organic cantaloupe

- Fresh juice of 1 organic blood orange (a standard orange is also fine)
- 1 tablespoon raw honey

Instructions:
Add coconut cream, cantaloupe, orange juice, and honey into a Vitamix blender and blend until it reaches a smooth consistency. Serve and eat immediately, or place in a glass jar and store in the refrigerator. Shelf life is 4 days.

10) **Raw Morning Liver Cleanse**

Step 1: **Tea base**
Ingredients:
- 2 tablespoons dandelion herb (buy loose leaf in bulk)
- 1 tablespoon milk thistle herb (buy loose in bulk)
- 2 cups filtered water

Instructions:
Add 2 tablespoons of dandelion and 1 tablespoon of milk thistle to a glass quart jar filled with 2 cups of water. Seal the jar. Place on the bare earth and steep in the sun for 8 hours. Strain the tea.

Step 2: **Tonic**
Ingredients:
- 1 organic pasture-raised raw egg
- ¼ cup organic grass-fed raw milk (or 2 teaspoons organic cold pressed olive oil)
- Fresh squeezed juice of 3 organic lemons
- 1 teaspoon organic raw apple cider vinegar

- Dash of organic cayenne pepper
- 2 tablespoons raw honey

Instructions:
Add egg, milk, lemon juice, apple cider vinegar, dash of cayenne pepper, and honey to the tea. Serve and eat immediately, or place in a glass jar and store in the refrigerator. Shelf life is 5 days.

11) <u>Raw Peanut Butter Weight Gain Smoothie</u>

Ingredients:
- 1½ cups organic grass-fed raw milk
- 1 organic pasture-raised raw egg
- 2 ripe organic bananas
- ½ cup raw wild jungle peanut butter (buy at a local Co-op)
- 1-2 tablespoons raw honey

Instructions:
Add milk, egg, bananas, peanut butter, and honey into a Vitamix blender and blend until it reaches a smooth consistency. Serve and eat immediately, or place in a glass jar and store in the refrigerator. Shelf life is 5 days.

12) <u>Raw Peach Cream Dream</u>

Ingredients:
- 1 cup organic grass-fed raw cream
- 2 organic pasture-raised raw eggs
- 2 pitted organic peaches
- 2 tablespoons raw honey

Instructions:
Add cream, eggs, peaches, and honey into a Vitamix blender and blend until ait reaches a smooth consistency. Serve and eat immediately, or place in a glass jar and store in the refrigerator. Shelf life is 5 days.

13) **Raw Carrot Creamsicle Juice**

Ingredients:
- 1½ cups fresh organic raw carrot juice
- 4 tablespoons organic grass-fed raw cream
- 1 tablespoon raw honey

Instructions:
Step 1:
Juice carrots in a juicer. Place juice into a 1 pint mason jar.

Step 2:
Add cream and honey to the mason jar and seal. Shake well. Serve and eat immediately, or place in a glass jar and store in the refrigerator. Shelf life is 3 days.

14) **Raw Orange Pomegranate Milkshake**

Ingredients:
- 2 cups organic grass-fed raw milk
- 2 organic pasture-raised raw eggs
- 1 whole peeled organic orange
- Fresh squeezed juice of 1 organic orange
- 4 teaspoons fresh organic pomegranate juice (when in season)
- ½ cup organic grass-fed raw cream
- ½ teaspoon raw vanilla bean powder
- 2 tablespoons raw honey

Instructions:
Add the milk, eggs, whole orange, juice of 1 orange, pomegranate juice, cream, vanilla bean powder, and honey into a Vitamix blender and blend until it reaches a smooth consistency. Serve and eat immediately, or place in a glass jar and store in the refrigerator. Shelf life is 5 days.

15) Raw Spirulina Milk

Ingredients:
- 2 cups organic grass-fed raw milk
- 2 organic pasture-raised raw eggs
- 3 heaping tablespoons raw cacao powder
- 1 teaspoon raw vanilla bean powder
- 1 teaspoon spirulina powder
- Pinch of cayenne (optional)
- 2 tablespoons raw honey

Instructions:
Add milk, eggs, cacao powder, vanilla bean powder, spirulina powder, and honey into a Vitamix blender and blend until it reaches a smooth consistency. Serve and eat immediately, or place in a glass jar and store in the refrigerator. Shelf life is 5 days.

16) Raw Egg Superfood Drink

Ingredients:
- 3 tablespoons organic grass-fed raw cream
- 3 organic pasture-raised raw eggs
- 1 teaspoon raw vanilla bean powder
- 1 teaspoon bee pollen
- 2 tablespoons raw honey

Instructions:

Add cream, eggs, vanilla bean powder, bee pollen, and honey into a Vitamix blender and blend until you it reaches a smooth consistency. Serve and eat immediately, or place in a glass jar and store in the refrigerator. Shelf life is 5 days.

17) **Iced Coffee Latte**

I don't drink coffee, however I like to enjoy this delicious treat at annual holiday parties.

Ingredients:
- 2 cups organic grass-fed raw milk
- 1 cup organic cold pressed coffee
- 2 organic pasture-raised raw egg yolks
- ½ cup organic grass-fed raw cream
- 1 teaspoon raw vanilla bean powder
- 3 tablespoons grade B maple syrup (not raw, and not usually recommended)

Instructions:

Add milk, cold pressed coffee, egg yolks, cream, vanilla bean powder, and maple syrup into a Vitamix blender and blend until it reaches a smooth consistency. Serve and eat immediately, or place in a glass jar and store in the refrigerator. Shelf life is 5 days.

18) **Raw Orange Vanilla Milkshake**

Ingredients:
- 2 cups organic grass-fed raw milk
- ½ cup organic grass-fed raw cream
- 1 organic pasture-raised raw egg
- ½ peeled organic orange

- 1/8 cup organic orange juice
- ½ teaspoon raw vanilla bean powder
- 1-2 tablespoons raw honey

Instructions:
Add milk, cream, egg, peeled orange, orange juice, vanilla bean powder, and honey into a Vitamix blender and blend until it reaches a smooth consistency. Serve and eat immediately, or place in a glass jar and store in the refrigerator. Shelf life is 5 days.

19) Raw Coconut Cream Peach Pudding

Ingredients:
- 1 cup fresh organic raw coconut cream (see raw condiments section)
- 3 fresh pitted organic peaches
- 1-2 tablespoons raw honey

Instructions:
Add coconut cream, peaches, and honey into a Vitamix blender and blend until it reaches a smooth consistency. Serve and eat immediately, or place in a glass jar and store in the refrigerator. Shelf life is 5 days.

20) Raw Raspberry Kefir

Ingredients:
- 2 cups organic grass-fed cow kefir
- 1 cup organic grass-fed raw cream
- 2 organic pasture-raised raw eggs
- 1 cup fresh organic raspberries
- 1 tablespoon raw honey

Instructions:
Add kefir, cream, eggs, raspberries, and honey into a Vitamix blender and blend until it reaches a smooth consistency. Serve and eat immediately, or place in a glass jar and store in the refrigerator. Shelf life is 5 days.

21) **Raw Sports Formula** (inspired by Aajonus Vonderplanitz)

Ingredients:
- 2 organic pasture-raised raw eggs
- 2 cups chopped fresh organic watermelon
- ½ peeled organic cucumber
- 2 medium sized organic tomatoes
- 3 tablespoons fresh organic lime juice
- 3 tablespoons fresh organic lemon juice
- 1 tablespoon raw organic apple cider vinegar
- 3 tablespoons fresh raw liquid whey (optional)
- 2 tablespoons raw honey

Instructions:
Add eggs, watermelon, cucumber, tomatoes, lime juice, lemon juice, apple cider vinegar, honey, and whey into a Vitamix blender and blend until it reaches a smooth consistency. Serve and eat immediately, or place in a glass jar and store in the refrigerator. Shelf life is 5 days.

22) **Raw Blackberry Butter Smoothie**

Ingredients:
- 2 cups organic grass-fed raw milk kefir
- 1 cup frozen organic blackberries (frozen from when in season)
- 6 tablespoons organic grass-fed raw butter (softened)

- 3 ripe organic bananas
- 5 pitted organic medjool dates

Instructions:
Add kefir, frozen blackberries, butter, ripe bananas, and dates into a Vitamix blender and blend until it reaches a smooth consistency. Serve and eat immediately, or place in a glass jar and store in the refrigerator. Shelf life is 5 days.

23) Raw Lemon Banana Smoothie

Ingredients:
- 2 ripe organic bananas
- 5 tablespoons organic grass-fed raw butter (softened)
- 1 organic pasture-raised raw egg
- Fresh squeezed juice of 3 organic lemons
- 1 tablespoon raw honey

Instructions:
Add bananas, butter, egg, fresh lemon juice, and honey to a Vitamix blender and blend until it reaches a smooth consistency. Serve and eat immediately, or store in a glass jar in your refrigerator. Shelf life is 5 days.

24) Raw Chia Cereal

Ingredients:
- 2 tablespoons chia seeds
- 1 cup organic grass-fed raw milk
- 1 sliced ripe banana

- 1 tablespoon raw cacao nibs
- 1-2 tablespoons raw honey

Step 1: **Soaking**
Instructions:
Put the chia seeds in a glass jar and fill the jar with 1 cup of milk. Place in the refrigerator over night until gelatinous.

Step 2: **Cereal**
Instructions:
Remove jar from the refrigerator, and shake. Add banana, cacao nibs, and honey to the jar. Shake the jar again. Serve and eat immediately, or store in a glass jar in your refrigerator. Shelf life is 5 days.

25) **Raw Brain Energizer**

Ingredients:
- 2 cups organic grass-fed raw milk
- 2 organic pasture-raised raw eggs
- 5 pitted organic medjool dates
- 1 tablespoon organic raw coconut oil
- 3 tablespoons raw cacao powder
- ½ teaspoon raw vanilla bean powder
- 1 tablespoon raw honey

Instructions:
Add milk, eggs, dates, coconut oil, cacao powder, vanilla bean powder, and honey into a Vitamix blender and blend until it reaches a smooth consistency. Serve and eat immediately, or store in a glass jar in your refrigerator. Shelf life is 5 days.

Twenty-One

RAW RED MEAT
(regenerative and anti-aging)

Steak tartare is simply raw meat and raw egg mixed together. Now, let's spice it up with these delicious and easy recipes.

<u>Tips</u>:

1. The best cuts of meat for making steak tartare are the lean cuts such as top sirloin, and the more expensive cut, filet mignon. Using a sharp knife, cut against the grain of the meat forming pieces that are 1/4 inch cubes or smaller.
2. One pound of ground meat makes 3 raw burgers.
3. Feel free to use either raw beef or raw bison in all of these recipes.

<u>All raw meats MUST be eaten fresh.</u>
<u>Do NOT eat any meat dish once it starts to smell or turn in color.</u>
<u>I suggest cooking the meat once it reaches this stage.</u>

1) <u>Raw Ground Bison Tartare</u>

<u>Ingredients</u>:
- 1 pound organic raw ground bison
- ¼ cup diced organic red onion
- 3 tablespoons organic fennel seeds
- 3 tablespoons fresh chopped organic sage
- 1 teaspoon diced organic red pepper
- 4 tablespoons organic cold pressed olive oil
- 2 tablespoons raw organic mustard (see raw mustard recipe in condiment section)
- 1 organic pasture-raised raw egg yolk

<u>Instructions</u>:
Add ground bison, red onion, fennel seeds, sage, red pepper, olive oil, and mustard into a glass bowl and mix together using your hands. Patty the meat into a burger shape while making space for an egg yolk to go on top. Place the egg yolk into the open space. Serve and eat immediately, or place in a glass jar and store in the refrigerator. Shelf life is 2 days.

If you haven't eaten the raw bison tartare within 2 days you can cook it lightly.

2) <u>Raw Bison Herb Burger</u>

<u>Ingredients</u>:
- 1 pound organic raw ground bison
- 1 small bunch chopped fresh organic basil
- 1 small bunch chopped fresh organic dill
- 4 tablespoons chopped fresh organic oregano

- 1 sliced medium organic tomato
- 4 tablespoons organic cold pressed olive oil
- ½ teaspoon organic cayenne pepper
- ½ teaspoon Himalayan salt
- 1 teaspoon raw honey
- 1 tablespoon raw mustard (topping: see raw mustard recipe in condiment section)
- 2 tablespoons raw sauerkraut (topping: from a local co-op)

Instructions:
Add ground bison, basil, dill, oregano, olive oil, cayenne pepper, salt and honey into a glass bowl and mix together using your hands. Patty the meat into a burger shape. Add a slice of tomato, mustard, and fermented sauerkraut on top. Serve and eat immediately, or place in a glass jar and store in the refrigerator. Shelf life is 2 days.

If you haven't eaten the raw bison burger within 2 days you can cook it lightly.

3) Raw Bison Tartare with Tartar Sauce

Step 1: Tartar Sauce
Ingredients:
- ½ cup homemade raw mayonnaise (see raw mayonnaise recipe in condiment section)
- 2 tablespoons pickle juice (use fermented pickle juice from homemade pickles: see pickle recipe in condiment section)
- 1 teaspoon fresh organic lemon juice
- 1 minced organic jalapeno
- ¼ teaspoon fresh organic garlic
- ½ teaspoon Himalayan salt

Instructions:
Add mayonnaise, pickle juice, lemon juice, jalapeno, garlic, and salt into a glass bowl and mix together using a wooden spoon.

Step 2: **Ground Bison**
Ingredients:
- 1 pound organic raw ground bison

Instructions:
Add ground bison and tartar sauce to a glass bowl and mix together using your hands. Serve and eat immediately, or place in a glass jar and store in the refrigerator. Shelf life is 2 days.

If you haven't eaten the raw bison tartare within 2 days you can cook it lightly.

4) Raw Beef Tenderloin Tartare

Ingredients:
- ½ pound organic raw beef tenderloin
- 2 tablespoons diced organic red onion
- ¼ bunch chopped fresh organic parsley
- 2 tablespoons organic cold pressed olive oil
- 1 teaspoon raw organic apple cider vinegar
- 1 teaspoon raw organic mustard (see raw mustard recipe in condiment section)
- 1 pinch organic cinnamon powder
- ½ teaspoon organic cayenne pepper
- 1 organic pasture-raised raw egg yolk
- 2 tablespoons organic wild Mediterranean capers in brine

Instructions:
Chop the meat into tiny pieces. Add meat, red onion, parsley, olive oil, apple cider vinegar, mustard, cinnamon, and cayenne pepper into a glass bowl and mix together using your hands. Patty the mixture into a burger shape while making space for an egg yolk to go on top. Place the raw egg yolk into the space, and place capers on top of the yolk. Serve and eat immediately, or place in a glass jar and store in the refrigerator. Shelf life is 2 days.

If you haven't eaten the raw beef tartare within 2 days you can cook it lightly.

5) **Raw Bison Garlic Burger**

Ingredients:
- ½ pound organic raw ground bison
- 2 tablespoons chopped organic red onion
- 2 minced organic garlic cloves
- 2 tablespoons organic grass-fed raw sour cream
- 2 tablespoons raw organic mustard (see raw mustard recipe in condiment section)
- ½ teaspoon organic cayenne pepper

Instructions:
Add bison, red onion, and garlic into a glass bowl and mix together using your hands. Patty the mixture into a burger shape. Top with sour cream, mustard, and sprinkle with cayenne. Serve and eat immediately, or place in a glass jar and store in the refrigerator. Shelf life is 2 days.

If you haven't eaten the raw bison burger within 2 days you can cook it lightly.

6) <u>Raw Avocado Bison Tartare</u>

<u>Ingredients</u>:
- 1 pound organic raw ground bison
- 3 tablespoons organic cold pressed olive oil
- 3 tablespoons diced organic red onion
- 1 handful chopped fresh organic cilantro
- 1 cubed organic avocado
- 1 small chopped organic roma tomato
- 2 chopped organic garlic cloves (optional)
- ½ teaspoon Himalayan salt

<u>Instructions</u>:
Add ground bison, olive oil, red onion, cilantro, avocado, tomato, garlic, and salt into a glass bowl and mix together using your hands. Serve and eat immediately, or place in a glass jar and store in the refrigerator. Shelf life is 2 days.

If you haven't eaten the raw bison tartare within 2 days you can cook it lightly.

7) <u>Raw Honey Mustard Bison Tartare</u>

<u>Ingredients</u>:
- ½ pound organic raw ground bison
- 2 tablespoons organic cold pressed olive oil
- 2 teaspoons organic raw mustard (see raw mustard recipe in condiment section)
- ½ teaspoon Himalayan salt
- 2 teaspoons raw honey

Instructions:
Add ground bison, olive oil, mustard, honey, and salt into a glass bowl and mix together using your hands. Serve and eat immediately, or place in a glass jar and store in the refrigerator. Shelf life is 2 days.

If you haven't eaten the raw bison tartare within 2 days you can cook it lightly.

8) Raw Beef Creamy Butter Tartare

Ingredients:
- 1 pound organic raw ground beef
- ¼ cup cubed organic grass-fed raw butter
- ¼ cup organic grass-fed raw cream (or sour cream)
- 1 teaspoon raw honey

Instructions:
Cut the butter into small square chunks. Add butter, ground beef, cream, and honey into a glass bowl and mix together using your hands. Serve and eat immediately, or place in a glass jar and store in the refrigerator. Shelf life is 2 days.

If you haven't eaten the raw beef tartare within 2 days you can cook it lightly

9) Raw Lemon Zest London Broil Strips

Ingredients:
- 1 pound organic raw London Broil (top round)
- 3 tablespoons finely chopped fresh organic parsley

- 4 tablespoons organic cold pressed olive oil
- 1-2 teaspoons fresh organic lemon zest (zest on a micro-plane)
- Fresh squeezed juice ½ organic lemon
- 1 teaspoon organic cayenne pepper
- 1 teaspoon Himalayan salt

Instructions:

Cut the steak into small sashimi style strips. Add steak strips, parsley, olive oil, lemon, lemon zest, cayenne pepper, and salt together into a glass bowl and mix together using your hands. Can be eaten sashimi style with chop sticks. Serve and eat immediately, or place in a glass jar and store in the refrigerator. Shelf life is 2 days.

If you haven't eaten the raw beef strips within 2 days you can cook them lightly.

10) **Raw kimchi Beef**

Ingredients:
- 1 pound organic raw ground beef
- 1 mashed organic avocado
- 1 teaspoon organic cayenne pepper
- ½ teaspoon Himalayan salt
- 1 teaspoon raw honey
- ¼ cup organic grass-fed raw butter chunks
- 1 cup kimchi (at a local co-op)

Instructions:

Add ground beef, kimchi, avocado, cayenne pepper, honey, and salt into a glass bowl and mix together using your hands. Mix in the chunks of butter, patty into a burger shape, and top with kimchi. Serve and eat immediately, or place in a glass jar and store in the refrigerator. Shelf life is 2 days.

If you haven't eaten the raw beef within 2 days you can cook it lightly.

11) Raw Hickory Beef

Step 1: Sauce
Ingredients:
- ½ cup chopped organic tomato
- 1 tablespoon organic cold pressed olive oil
- ½ cup sun dried tomatoes (soak for 1 hour in filtered water)
- ¼ cup chopped organic fresh basil
- ¼ cup pitted organic medjool dates
- ¼ cup chopped organic red onion
- 1 tablespoon chopped organic jalapeno
- 2 teaspoons crushed organic garlic
- ½ tablespoon raw honey

Instructions:
Add tomato, olive oil, sun dried tomatoes, basil, dates, red onion, jalapeno, garlic, and honey into a Vitamix blender and blend until it reaches a smooth consistency.

Step 2: Beef
Ingredients:
- 1 pound organic raw ground beef
- 1 cup pre-blended sauce
- ¼ cup chopped organic red onion

- ¼ teaspoon organic curry powder
- 2 tablespoons organic cold pressed olive oil
- 2 teaspoons chopped fresh organic oregano
- ¼ pound organic grass-fed raw butter cut into small chunks

Instructions:

Add ground beef, sauce, red onion, curry powder, olive oil, and oregano into a glass bowl and mix together using your hands. Mix in the small chunks of butter. Serve and eat immediately, or place in a glass jar and store in the refrigerator. Shelf life is 2 days.

If you haven't eaten the raw beef within 2 days you can cook it lightly.

12) Raw Bison Cheese Burger

Step 1: **Burger**
Ingredients:
- 1 pound organic raw ground bison
- 1 finely chopped organic carrot
- 1 finely chopped organic celery stalk
- ¼ finely chopped organic red onion

Instructions:

Add ground bison, carrots, celery, and red onion into a glass bowl and mix together using your hands. Patty into burger shapes.

Step 2: **Raw Cheese Sauce**
Ingredients:
- ½ pound organic grass-fed raw cheese (allow to soften for several hours on a counter)

- 1 organic pasture-raised raw egg
- 3 tablespoons organic cold pressed olive oil
- 1 finely chopped organic jalapeno
- 1 tablespoon fresh squeezed organic lemon juice
- ½ teaspoon Himalayan salt

Instructions:
Add cheese, egg, olive oil, jalapeno, lemon juice, and salt into a food processor and mix until it reaches a smooth consistency.

Step 3: **Wrap**
- 1 head organic red leaf lettuce (or any soft lettuce)
- 1 sliced tomato
- 1 tablespoon raw mustard

Instructions:
Place the red leaf lettuce onto a cutting board, put burger patty in the middle of the lettuce, spread the cheese sauce onto the patty, and layer with mustard and fresh tomato. Wrap the lettuce around the burger. Serve and eat immediately, or place in a glass jar and store in the refrigerator. Shelf life is 2 days.

If you haven't eaten the raw burger within 2 days you can cook it lightly.

13) **Flat Iron Steak**

Ingredients:
- ½ pound tiny cubed organic raw flat iron steak
- 2 tablespoons organic cold pressed olive oil
- Dash organic cayenne pepper

- 2 tablespoons organic micro greens (optional)
- ¼ teaspoon Himalayan Salt

<u>Instructions</u>:
Add steak, olive oil, cayenne pepper, and salt into a glass bowl and mix together using your hands. Top with the micro greens. Serve and eat immediately, or place in a glass jar and store in the refrigerator. Shelf life is 2 days.

If you haven't eaten the raw steak within 2 days you can cook it lightly.

Twenty-Two

RAW CHICKEN CEVICHE
(your new favorite)

Ceviche is a great way to introduce yourself to the raw paleo diet. It's easy, tasty, and has less of the "raw" feeling.

Directions:

1) Cutting the chicken
Every recipe calls for 3 raw chicken breasts to be cut into 1/4 inch cubes or smaller. This will give you the two cups of "cold cooked" chicken required for the recipes.

2) "Cold Cooking" the Chicken in Fresh Squeezed Lemon Juice
These recipes require 48 hours of "cold cooking" in fresh lemon juice. Place the chicken cubes into a 1/2 gallon glass jar. Add enough lemon juice to completely cover the raw chicken cubes. Place a lid on the jar and allow it to sit in the refrigerator for 48 hours.

3) <u>Draining the Lemon Juice from the Chicken</u>
Squeeze the lemon juice thoroughly out of the chicken. This makes the ceviche less lemony and more palatable.

Remove the chicken from the glass jar and strain through a nut milk bag, cheese-cloth, or anything finely meshed to get the lemon thoroughly out. Alternatively, you can squeeze the chicken firmly with your hands over a strainer.

4) <u>Hand-Cutting the Herbs</u>
I've found that hand-cutting the herbs offer a richer flavor than when I've used a food processor. The fresher the herbs, the better the flavor will be.

5) <u>Side of Avocado</u>
The chicken ceviche dishes are delicious on their own, however they also go well with slices of avocado and fermented vegetables.

1) **Raw Chicken Curry Ceviche**

<u>Ingredients:</u>
- 2 cups "cold cooked" organic pasture-raised raw chicken (see directions)
- 1 organic pasture-raised raw egg yolk
- ¼ cup organic grass-fed raw cream
- 6 tablespoons organic cold pressed olive oil
- 2 tablespoons organic apple cider vinegar
- 2 tablespoons organic curry powder
- 1 small minced organic garlic clove
- 1-2 chopped organic tomatoes
- 1 teaspoon raw honey
- ¼ teaspoon Himalayan salt

Instructions:

Add "cold cooked" chicken, egg yolk, cream, olive oil, apple cider vinegar, curry powder, and garlic into a glass bowl and mix together using your hands. Add tomatoes, honey, and Himalayan salt. Serve and eat immediately, or place in a glass jar and store in the refrigerator. Shelf life is 4 days.

2) Raw Chicken Cheddar Ceviche

Ingredients:
- 2 cups "cold cooked" organic pasture-raised raw chicken (see directions)
- 1 cup organic grass-fed raw cheddar cheese (allow to soften on counter for a few hours prior to use)
- ½ cup diced organic red onion
- 1 chopped organic jalapeno
- 1 tablespoon organic raw apple cider vinegar
- Fresh squeezed juice of 1 organic lemon
- ½ teaspoon Himalayan salt

Instructions:
Step 1: **Sauce**
Add softened cheese, red onion, jalapeno, apple cider vinegar, lemon juice, and salt into a food processor and mix until it reaches a smooth consistency.

Step 2: **Chicken**
Add sauce and "cold cooked" chicken into a glass bowl and mix together using your hands. Serve and eat immediately, or place in a glass jar and store in the refrigerator. Shelf life is 4 days.

3) <u>Raw Chicken Garlic Ceviche</u>

<u>Ingredients</u>:
- 2 cups "cold cooked" organic pasture-raised raw chicken (see directions)
- ½ cup organic grass-fed raw white cheddar cheese (allow to soften on counter for a few hours prior to use)
- 1 organic pasture-raised raw egg yolk
- 3 tablespoons chopped fresh organic oregano
- 2 minced organic garlic cloves
- 1 tablespoon organic raw apple cider vinegar
- 1 tablespoon raw honey

<u>Instructions</u>:
<u>Step 1</u>: **Sauce**
Add softened cheese, egg yolk, garlic, apple cider vinegar, and honey into a Vitamix blender and blend until it reaches a smooth consistency.

<u>Step 2</u>: **Chicken**
Add sauce and "cold cooked" chicken into a glass bowl and mix together using your hands. Top with fresh oregano. Serve and eat immediately, or place in a glass jar and store in the refrigerator. Shelf life is 4 days.

4) <u>Raw Chicken Basil Cream Ceviche</u>

<u>Ingredients</u>:
- 2 cups "cold cooked" organic pasture-raised raw chicken (see directions)
- 1/3 cup organic grass-fed raw cream
- 1 handful chopped fresh organic basil

- 1 mashed organic avocado
- 1 minced organic jalapeno
- 2 tablespoons chopped organic green onion
- 1 teaspoon raw honey
- ½ teaspoon organic cayenne pepper
- ½ teaspoon Himalayan salt

Instructions:

Add "cold cooked" chicken, cream, basil, avocado, jalapeno, green onion, honey, cayenne pepper, and salt into a glass bowl and mix together using your hands. Serve and eat immediately, or place in a glass jar and store in the refrigerator. Shelf life is 4 days.

5) **Raw Chicken Herb Ceviche**

Ingredients:
- 2 cups "cold cooked" organic pasture-raised raw chicken (see directions)
- 2 tablespoons organic grass-fed raw cream
- 3 tablespoons chopped fresh organic parsley
- 4 tablespoons chopped fresh organic dill
- 2 tablespoons chopped organic red onion
- 2 tablespoons organic cold pressed olive oil
- ½ teaspoon Himalayan salt

Instructions:

Add "cold cooked" chicken, cream, parsley, dill, red onion, olive oil, and salt into a glass bowl and mix together using your hands. Serve and eat immediately, or place in a glass jar and store in the refrigerator. Shelf life is 4 days.

6) Raw Sweet and Spicy Chicken Salad

Ingredients:
- 2 cups "cold cooked" organic pasture-raised raw chicken (see directions)
- ¼ cup organic grass-fed raw cream
- 3 tablespoons chopped fresh organic mint leaves
- 4 tablespoons organic cold pressed olive oil
- Fresh squeezed juice of 1 organic orange
- 1 teaspoon organic cayenne pepper
- ¼ teaspoon Himalayan salt

Instructions:
Add "cold cooked" chicken, cream, mint leaves, olive oil, orange juice, cayenne pepper, and salt into a glass bowl and mix together using your hands. Serve and eat immediately, or place in a glass jar and store in the refrigerator. Shelf life is 4 days.

7) Raw Barbeque Chicken Ceviche

Ingredients:
- 2 cups "cold cooked" organic pasture-raised raw chicken (see directions)
- 3 tablespoons organic grass-fed raw cream
- 3 tablespoons chopped sun dried tomatoes (soak in filtered water for 2 hours)
- 3 tablespoons chopped organic red onion
- 1 chopped organic tomato
- 2 minced organic garlic cloves
- 2 tablespoons organic cold pressed olive oil
- 1 teaspoon organic raw apple cider vinegar

- 2 teaspoons organic cumin powder
- ½ teaspoon organic cayenne pepper
- ½ teaspoon Himalayan salt

Instructions:
Add "cold cooked" chicken, sun dried tomato, red onion, tomato, garlic, olive oil, apple cider vinegar, cumin powder, cayenne pepper, and salt into a glass bowl and mix together using your hands. Drizzle cream on top of the ceviche. Serve and eat immediately, or place in a glass jar and store in the refrigerator. Shelf life is 4 days.

8) Raw Hawaiian Chicken Ceviche

Ingredients:
- 2 cups "cold cooked" organic pasture-raised raw chicken (see directions)
- ¼ cup organic grass-fed raw cream
- 1 cup chopped organic pineapple
- 2 finely chopped organic celery stalks
- ¼ cup chopped fresh organic tarragon
- ¼ cup chopped fresh organic mint
- 2 tablespoons organic cold pressed olive oil
- 1 tablespoon raw honey
- ½ teaspoon Himalayan salt
- ½ cup raw coconut shreds (optional)

Instructions:
Add "cold cooked" chicken, cream, pineapple, celery, tarragon, mint, olive oil, honey, and salt into a glass bowl and mix together using your hands. Sprinkle coconut shreds on top of the ceviche. Serve and eat immediately, or place in a glass jar and store in the refrigerator. Shelf life is 4 days.

9) Raw Tomato Chicken Ceviche

Ingredients:
- 2 cups "cold cooked" organic pasture-raised raw chicken (see directions)
- 1 cup chopped organic tomatoes
- 1 bunch chopped organic green onion
- ¼ cup organic cold pressed olive oil
- ½ teaspoon Himalayan salt

Instructions:
Add "cold cooked" chicken, tomatoes, green onion, olive oil, and salt into a glass bowl and mix together using your hands. Serve and eat immediately, or place in a glass jar and store in the refrigerator. Shelf life is 4 days.

10) Raw Thanksgiving Chicken Salad

Ingredients:
- 2 cups "cold cooked" organic pasture-raised raw chicken (see directions)
- ¼ cup homemade raw mayonnaise (see raw mayonnaise recipe in condiment section)
- 2 finely chopped organic celery stalks
- 3 tablespoons chopped organic white onion
- 2 tablespoons organic wild Mediterranean capers in brine
- 3 tablespoons chopped fresh organic sage
- ¼ teaspoon organic cayenne pepper
- Dash Himalayan salt

Instructions:
Add "cold cooked" chicken, mayonnaise, celery, white onion, capers, sage, cayenne pepper, and salt into a glass bowl and mix together using your

hands. Serve and eat immediately, or place in a glass jar and store in the refrigerator. Shelf life is 4 days.

11) <u>Raw Country Chicken Ceviche</u>

This recipe is different from the others because you are required to "cold cook" the chicken in a marinade that you will make. This is instead of "cold cooking" the chicken in lemon juice as per the other chicken recipes.

<u>Step 1</u>: **Making the Marinade**
<u>Ingredients</u>:
- ½ cup organic raw apple cider vinegar
- ½ cup fresh squeezed organic lemon juice
- ½ cup organic cold pressed olive oil

<u>Instructions</u>:
Add apple cider vinegar, lemon juice, and olive oil into a Vitamix blender and blend until it reaches a smooth consistency.

<u>Step 2</u>: **Marinating the Chicken**
<u>Ingredients</u>:
3 organic pasture-raised raw chicken breasts

<u>Instructions</u>:
Cut the chicken into 1/4 inch cubes or smaller, place into a glass jar, cover completely with the marinade from step 1, and seal the jar. Allow the chicken to marinate in this marinade for 48 hours in the refrigerator.

<u>Step 3</u>: **Making the Chicken Ceviche**
<u>Ingredients</u>:
- 2 cups marinated chicken (from step 2)
- 2 finely chopped organic celery stalks

- ½ peeled, finely chopped organic cucumber
- 1 finely chopped organic carrot
- ¼ cup chopped organic scallions
- 1 teaspoon minced organic garlic
- 1 tablespoon chopped organic jalapeno
- 1 tablespoon fresh squeezed organic lime juice
- 1 teaspoon raw honey
- ¼ teaspoon Himalayan Salt

Instructions:

Add marinated chicken, celery, cucumber, carrot, scallions, garlic, jalapeno, lime juice, honey, and salt into a glass bowl and mix together using your hands. Serve and eat immediately, or place in a glass jar and store in the refrigerator. Shelf life is 5 days.

Note: To spice up this recipe you can also make *Cayenne Country Chicken* by adding 1 teaspoon of organic cayenne pepper to the finished dish.

Twenty-Three

RAW FISH CEVICHE
(spice up your life)

Ceviche is raw fish that's been "cold cooked" in fresh squeezed lemon juice. It's usually mixed with organic vegetables and herbs. To make raw fish ceviche it's best to use a mild boneless filet of white fish such as Pacific sole/flounder. However opah, halibut, cod, tuna, and various shell fish can also be used. Generally, sole will have less fishy taste and hold up better in lemon juice.

Directions:

1) Cutting the Fish
Every recipe calls for 1 pound of raw fish to be cut into 1/4 inch cubes or smaller. Remove the skin, bones, or mushy side trim. If the fish smells fishy I suggest first rinsing in cold water.

2) "Cold Cooking" the Fish in Fresh Squeezed Lemon Juice
These recipes require 24 hours of "cold cooking" the fish in fresh lemon juice. Place the fish cubes into a 1/2 gallon glass jar. Add enough lemon

juice to completely cover the raw fish cubes. Place a lid on the jar and allow it to sit in the refrigerator for 24 hours.

3) <u>Draining the Lemon Juice from the Fish</u>
Squeeze the lemon juice thoroughly out of the fish. This makes the ceviche less lemony and more palatable. Remove the fish from the glass jar
and strain through a nut milk bag, cheesecloth, or anything finely meshed
to get the lemon thoroughly out. Alternatively, you can squeeze the fish
firmly with your hands over a strainer.

4) <u>Hand-Cutting the Herbs</u>
I have found that hand-cutting the herbs offer a richer flavor than when I've
used a food processor. The fresher the herbs, the better the flavor will be.

5) <u>Side of Avocado</u>
The fish ceviche dishes are delicious on their own however they also go
well with slices of avocado and fermented vegetables.

6) <u>Ginger juice</u>
Juice the ginger in a home juicer, or grate on a microplane or cheese
grater, and then squeeze through a metal tea strainer.

1) Raw Tomato Cod Ceviche
This recipe is different from the others because you are required to marinate the fish in a marinade that you will make, instead of soaking in lemon
juice as per the other fish recipes.

<u>Step 1</u>: **Making the Marinade**
<u>Ingredients</u>:
- 1 cup organic raw apple cider vinegar
- ¼ cup organic cold pressed olive oil

Instructions:
Place the apple cider vinegar and olive oil in a glass pint jar and shake until well mixed.

Step 2: **Making the Ceviche**
Ingredients:
- 1 pound raw wild cod
- 2 tablespoons organic cold pressed olive oil
- 1 cup chopped organic cherry tomatoes
- ½ teaspoon organic cayenne pepper
- ½ teaspoon Himalayan salt

Instructions:
Cut the fish into 1/4 inch cubes and place into a glass quart jar. Add the marinade into the jar until the fish completely covered. Seal the jar and place in the refrigerator for 24 hours.

After 24 hours of marinating, leave all of the marinade in the jar, add tomatoes, olive oil, cayenne pepper, and salt to the jar. Shake the quart jar well. Serve and eat immediately, or place in a glass jar and store in the refrigerator. Shelf life is 4 days.

2) **Raw Halibut Ceviche**

Ingredients:
- 1 pound "cold cooked" raw wild halibut (see directions)
- 1 small chopped organic red pepper
- ½ diced organic jalapeno
- 4 tablespoons chopped organic red onion
- 2 chopped organic tomatoes
- ½ cubed organic avocado

- 1 bunch chopped fresh organic cilantro
- ½ teaspoon Himalayan salt

Instructions:
Add "cold cooked" and drained fish, red pepper, jalapeno, red onion, to-matoes, avocado, cilantro, and salt into a glass bowl and mix together us-ing your hands. Serve and eat immediately, or place in a glass jar and store in the refrigerator. Shelf life is 4 days.

3) Raw Sweet Creamy Sole

Ingredients:
- 1 pound "cold cooked" raw wild sole (see directions)
- 3 tablespoons organic grass-fed raw cream
- 1½ chopped organic tomatoes
- 2 tablespoons chopped organic red onion
- ½ mashed organic avocado
- 1 handful chopped organic fresh dill
- 1 tablespoon organic raw mustard (see raw mustard recipe in condiment section)
- 1 teaspoon raw honey
- ½ teaspoon Himalayan salt

Instructions:
Add "cold cooked" and drained fish, cream, tomatoes, red onion, avocado, dill, mustard, honey, and salt into a glass bowl and mix together using your hands. Serve and eat immediately, or place in a glass jar and store in the refrigerator. Shelf life is 4 days.

4) Raw Spicy Seafood Melody
Avoid all shrimps from Asia and Gulf of Mexico.

Ingredients:
- ¼ pound "cold cooked" raw wild shrimp (see directions)
- ¼ pound "cold cooked" raw wild crab (see directions)
- ¼ pound "cold cooked" raw wild lobster (see directions)
- 1 chopped organic tomato
- ½ cubed organic avocado
- 2 tablespoons chopped organic red onion
- ¼ tablespoon chopped organic habanero
- 1 bunch chopped fresh organic cilantro
- 2 tablespoons organic cold pressed olive oil
- ½ teaspoon Himalayan salt

Instructions:
Add "cold cooked" and <u>drained</u> seafood, tomato, avocado, red onion, habanero, cilantro, olive oil, and salt into a glass bowl and mix together using your hands. Serve and eat immediately, or place in a glass jar and store in the refrigerator. Shelf life is 4 days.

5) <u>Raw Lime Ceviche</u>

Ingredients:
- ½ pound "cold cooked" raw wild flounder (see directions, however use lime instead of lemon)
- ¼ peeled and cubed organic cucumber
- ½ thinly sliced organic white onion
- 1 teaspoon raw honey (optional)
- ¼ teaspoon Himalayan salt

Instructions:
Add "cold cooked" and <u>drained</u> fish, cucumber, onion, honey, and salt into a glass bowl and mix together using your hands. Serve and eat

immediately, or place in a glass jar and store in the refrigerator. Shelf life is 4 days.

6) Raw Poke Tuna Tartare

Ingredients:
- 1 pound "cold cooked" raw wild yellowfin tuna (see directions)
- 3 tablespoons chopped organic green onion
- 2 tablespoons organic ginger juice (grated on a microplane and squeeze)
- 3 tablespoons organic cold pressed olive oil
- ¼ teaspoon organic lemon juice
- ¼ teaspoon organic cayenne pepper
- ¼ teaspoon Himalayan salt

Instructions:
Add "cold cooked" and drained fish, green onion, ginger juice, olive oil, lemon, cayenne pepper, and salt into a glass bowl and mix together using your hands. Serve and eat immediately, or place in a glass jar and store in the refrigerator. Shelf life is 4 days.

7) Raw Spicy Fish Ceviche

Ingredients:
- 1 pound "cold cooked" raw wild halibut (see directions)
- ½ cup chopped organic tomato
- ¼ cup chopped organic red onion
- ¼ cup chopped fresh organic dill
- 1-2 tablespoons minced organic jalapeno

- 1 tablespoon fresh organic lime zest (zest on a microplane)
- 2 tablespoons organic cold pressed olive oil
- 1 tablespoon raw honey
- ½ teaspoon cayenne pepper
- ½ teaspoon Himalayan Salt

Instructions:
Add "cold cooked" and <u>drained</u> fish, tomato, red onion, dill, jalapeno, lime zest, olive oil, honey, cayenne pepper, and salt into a glass bowl and mix together using your hands. Serve and eat immediately, or place in a glass jar and store in the refrigerator. Shelf life is 4 days.

8) <u>Raw Mango Fish Ceviche</u>

Ingredients:
- 1 pound "cold cooked" raw wild flounder (see directions)
- ½ cup chopped organic tomato
- ¼ cup chopped organic red onion
- ½ cup chopped organic mango
- ½ cup chopped organic cilantro
- 2 teaspoons grated organic ginger (grate on a microplane)
- 3 tablespoons organic cold pressed olive oil
- 1 tablespoon raw honey

Instructions:
Add "cold cooked" and <u>drained</u> fish, tomato, red onion, mango, cilantro, ginger, olive oil, and honey into a glass bowl and mix together using your hands. Serve and eat immediately, or place in a glass jar and store in the refrigerator. Shelf life is 4 days.

9) Raw Sweet Ginger Lime Ceviche

Ingredients:
- 1 pound "cold cooked" raw wild flounder (see directions)
- ½ cup chopped organic tomato
- 1/8 cup chopped organic red onion
- ¼ cup chopped fresh organic cilantro
- 3 tablespoons organic cold pressed olive oil
- 1½ teaspoons grated ginger (grate on a microplane)
- 1 teaspoon organic fresh lime zest (zest on microplane)
- 2 tablespoons raw honey

Instructions:
Add "cold cooked" and drained fish, tomato, red onion, cilantro, olive oil, ginger, lime zest, and honey into a glass bowl and mix together using your hands. Serve and eat immediately, or place in a glass jar and store in the refrigerator. Shelf life is 4 days.

10) Raw Tuna Salad Ceviche

Ingredients:
- 1 pound "cold cooked" raw wild tuna (see directions)
- ½ cup raw mayonnaise (see raw mayonnaise recipe in condiment section)
- ¼ cup organic grass-fed raw cream
- 1 finely chopped organic celery stalk
- ¼ cup finely chopped pickles (see pickle recipe in condiment section)
- ½ cup chopped apples into tiny squares
- 4 tablespoons organic raw mustard (see raw mustard recipe in condiment section)

Instructions:
Add "cold cooked" and <u>drained</u> fish, mayonnaise, cream, celery, pickles, apples, and mustard into a glass bowl and mix together using your hands. Serve and eat immediately, or place in a glass jar and store in the refrigerator. Shelf life is 4 days.

11) Raw Spicy Garlic Shrimp Ceviche

Step1: **Spicy Garlic Sauce**
Ingredients:
- ½ cup chopped organic tomato
- 1 teaspoon grated ginger (grate on a microplane)
- ¼ cup organic cold pressed olive oil
- 1 teaspoon organic lime zest (zest on a microplane)
- 1 tablespoon organic raw apple cider vinegar
- 1 inch minced organic jalapeno
- 4 minced organic garlic cloves
- 1 tablespoon raw honey

Instructions:
Add tomatoes, ginger, olive oil, lime zest, apple cider vinegar, jalapeno, garlic, and honey into a Vitamix blender and blend until it reaches a smooth consistency.

Step 2: **Ceviche**
Ingredients:
- 1 pound "cold cooked" raw wild shrimp (see directions)
- ½ cup spicy garlic sauce
- ¼ cup chopped organic fresh dill

Instructions:

Add "cold cooked" and <u>drained</u> fish, spicy garlic sauce, and dill into a glass bowl and mix together using your hands. Serve and eat immediately, or place in a glass jar and store in the refrigerator. Shelf life is 4 days.

Twenty-Four

1) <u>Raw Liver Pate</u> (inspired by Anthony Farano)

<u>Step 1</u>: **Soaking the Liver**
<u>Ingredients</u>:
- ½ cup organic grass-fed raw bison liver (or beef liver)
- ½ cup organic grass-fed raw milk

<u>Instructions</u>:
Cut the raw liver into ½ inch cubes and place into a glass bowl. Add milk into the bowl and allow the liver to soak for 20 minutes on a counter. Rinse the liver using filtered water. Squeeze out any extra surface water with your hands.

<u>Step 2</u>: **Blending the Pate**
<u>Ingredients</u>:
- ½ cup soaked organic grass-fed raw bison liver (or beef liver)
- ¾ cup organic grass-fed butter (softened)

- 2 organic pasture-raised raw eggs
- 2 tablespoons chopped organic red onion
- 3 inches grated organic ginger root (grate on a microplane)
- 3 inches grated organic turmeric root (grate on a microplane)
- 2 tablespoons organic raw mustard (see raw mustard recipe in condiment section)
- 1 teaspoon organic raw apple cider vinegar
- 1-2 tablespoons raw honey
- ½ teaspoon Himalayan salt

Instructions:
Add liver, butter, eggs, red onion, ginger, turmeric, mustard, apple cider vinegar, honey, and salt into a Vitamix blender and blend until it reaches a smooth consistency. This may take up to five minutes to blend completely. Serve and eat immediately, or place in a glass jar and store in the refrigerator. Shelf life is 1 week.

2) **Raw Chicken Liver Smoothie**

Ingredients:
- 1 organic grass-fed raw chicken liver
- 1½ cups organic grass-fed raw milk
- ¼ cup organic grass-fed raw cream
- 1 organic pasture-raised raw egg
- ¾ cup fresh organic blueberries
- 4 fresh organic strawberries
- 2 tablespoons raw honey
- 1 cup ice

Instructions:
Add liver, milk, cream, egg, blueberries, strawberries, honey, and ice into a Vitamix blender and blend until it reaches a smooth consistency. Serve

and eat immediately, or place in a glass jar and store in the refrigerator. Shelf life is 4 days.

3) <u>Raw Heart Carpaccio</u>

<u>Ingredients</u>:
- ½ pound organic grass-fed raw bison heart (or beef heart)
- 1 small thinly sliced organic white onion
- Drizzle organic cold pressed olive oil
- Shake organic cayenne pepper
- Shake Himalayan Salt

<u>Instructions</u>:
Cut the heart into thin slices and place on a plate. Top with thinly sliced white onion, drizzle of olive oil, dash cayenne pepper, and some Himalayan salt. Serve and eat immediately, or place in a glass jar and store in the refrigerator. Shelf life is 4 days.

Twenty-Five

Raw Bone Marrow
(rejuvenating delicacies)

I t's preferable to use fresh (never frozen) organic grass-fed marrow bones. These bones are obtainable from a local butcher shop or health food market. If you can't find fresh marrow bones, then frozen bones are fine.

1) Raw Strawberry Marrow Pudding

Step1: **Blending the Pudding**
Ingredients:
- ¼ cup chopped organic grass-fed raw bone marrow
- 1 cup organic fresh strawberries
- 3 tablespoons organic grass-fed raw butter (softened)
- 1 organic pasture-raised raw egg
- 1 tablespoon raw honey

Instructions:
Scrape the raw marrow from the inside of the bone. Add marrow, strawberries, butter, egg, and honey into a Vitamix blender and

blend until it reaches a very smooth consistency. If the mixture becomes chunky or gritty just keep blending until it reaches a smooth consistency.

Step 2: **Adding the Cream**
Ingredients:
- ½ cup organic grass-fed raw cream

Instructions:
Add cream to the ingredients in the Vitamix blender, and blend slowly on a low speed for 3-5 seconds. Blend for the shortest amount possible until the ingredients are mixed well. Serve and eat immediately, or place in a glass jar and store in the refrigerator. Shelf life is 5 days.

Note: If you blend the cream for too long it will turn into butter, which is not a good consistency for the pudding.

2) Raw Vanilla Marrow Custard

Ingredients:
- ¼ cup chopped organic grass-fed raw bone marrow
- 3 tablespoons organic grass-fed raw butter (softened)
- 2 organic pasture-raised raw eggs
- 2 tablespoons organic raw coconut oil (soften in a bowl of warm water)
- 1 teaspoon raw vanilla bean powder
- 1 tablespoon raw honey
- Pinch of Himalayan salt (optional)

Instructions:
Scrape the raw marrow from the inside of the bone. Add marrow, butter, eggs, coconut oil, vanilla bean powder, and honey into a Vitamix blender and blend until it reaches a smooth consistency. If the mixture becomes

chunky or gritty just keep blending until it reaches a smooth consistency. Serve and eat immediately, or place in a glass jar and store in the refrigerator. Shelf life is 5 days.

3) <u>Raw Creamy Chocolate Marrow Mousse</u>

<u>Step 1</u>: **Blending the Mousse**
<u>Ingredients</u>:
- ¼ cup chopped organic grass-fed raw bone marrow
- 3 Tablespoons organic grass-fed raw butter (softened)
- 2 organic pasture-raised raw eggs
- 3 tablespoons raw cacao powder
- 1 tablespoon raw honey

<u>Instructions</u>:
Scrape the raw marrow from the inside of the bone. Add marrow, butter, eggs, cacao powder, and honey into a Vitamix blender and blend until it reaches a smooth consistency. If the mixture becomes chunky or gritty just keep blending until it reaches a smooth consistency. Serve and eat immediately, or place in a glass jar and store in the refrigerator. Shelf life is 5 days.

<u>Step 2</u>: **Adding the Cream**
<u>Ingredients</u>:
- ½ cup organic grass-fed raw cream

<u>Instructions</u>:
Add cream to the ingredients in the Vitamix blender, and blend slowly on a low speed for 3-5 seconds. Blend for the shortest amount possible until the ingredients are mixed well. Serve and eat immediately, or place in a glass jar and store in the refrigerator. Shelf life is 5 days.

Note: If you blend the cream for too long it will turn into butter, which is not a good consistency for the pudding.

4) Raw Orange Cream Marrow Mousse

Step 1: **Blending the Mousse**
Ingredients:
- ¼ cup chopped organic grass-fed raw bone marrow
- 3 Tablespoons organic grass-fed butter(softened)
- ¼ cup fresh squeezed organic orange juice
- 1 organic pasture-raised raw egg
- 2 tablespoons raw honey

Instructions:
Scrape the raw marrow from the inside of the bone. Add marrow, egg, orange juice, and honey into a Vitamix blender and blend until it reaches a smooth consistency. If the mixture becomes chunky or gritty just keep blending until it reaches a smooth consistency.

Step 2: **Adding the Cream**
Ingredients:
- ½ cup organic grass-fed raw cream

Instructions:
Add cream to the ingredients in the Vitamix blender, and blend slowly on a low speed for 3-5 seconds. Blend for the shortest amount possible until the ingredients are mixed well. Serve and eat immediately, or place in a glass jar and store in the refrigerator. Shelf life is 5 days.

Note: If you blend the cream for too long it will turn into butter, which is not a good consistency for the pudding.

5) <u>Raw Pineapple Marrow Pudding</u>

<u>Ingredients</u>:
- ¼ cup chopped organic grass-fed raw bone marrow
- ½ chopped organic pineapple
- 5 tablespoons organic grass-fed raw butter (softened)
- 1 organic pasture-raised raw egg
- 1 tablespoon raw honey

<u>Instructions</u>:
Scrape the raw marrow from the inside of the bone. Add marrow, pineapple, butter, egg, and honey into a Vitamix blender and blend until it reaches a smooth consistency. If the mixture becomes chunky or gritty just keep blending until it reaches a smooth consistency. Serve and eat immediately, or place in a glass jar and store in the refrigerator. Shelf life is 5 days.

Twenty-Six

RAW PALEO BEAUTY
(do-it-yourself skincare)

I recommend that you put on your skin only that which you would also eat. Skin products will absorb directly into your bloodstream, and if not made from food will contribute toxins to your body. The ingredients used in typical personal care products can disrupt hormones, impede digestion, alter brain function, disrupt reproductive health, and much more.

If someone is ill, I especially recommend that they eliminate all personal care products that aren't made from food. Would you eat the shampoo that's in your shower right now?

1) __Raw Coconut Cream Soap__
This recipe makes a great antibacterial soap that will allow your skin to stay soft all day long. Did you know that fifty years ago most soaps contained coconut cream?

Ingredients:
- Fermented organic raw coconut cream (see coconut cream recipe in condiments section)

Instructions:
Fermented raw coconut cream is made by simply allowing fresh coconut cream to naturally ferment in a glass jar while in the refrigerator. This usually takes 1-3 weeks. Take the glass jar into the shower and use instead of your regular soap.

Note: The floor of your shower may become slippery, so be very careful.

2) Raw Butter Soap

Ingredients:
- 4 tablespoons organic grass-fed raw butter

My story:
Once while traveling I forgot to bring soap, but sure enough I had raw butter with me. I decided to bring it into the shower and "buttered me up" with it. Be sure to rinse afterwards. I had a slight buttery smell but my skin was so soft and felt protected.

3) Natural Deodorant

Ingredients:
- 2 tablespoons organic raw coconut oil (soften in a bowl of warm water)
- 2 tablespoons arrow root powder
- 2 tablespoons baking soda
- 5 drops lemongrass essential oil

Instructions:
Add equal parts of coconut oil, arrow root powder, and baking soda into a glass bowl and mix together until combined well. Stir in 5 drops of lemongrass essential oil for a pleasant smell. Place in a 4oz glass jar and seal. Shelf life is 6 months at room temperature.

4) **Raw Lemon Deodorant**

Ingredients:
- Fresh squeezed juice of 1 organic lemon

Instructions:
Dip your fingers into the lemon juice and dab under your arms.

5) **Raw Odor Removal Bath**

Ingredients:
- 1-2 cups organic raw apple cider vinegar

Instructions:
Fill a bath with hot water. Add 1-2 cups of apple cider vinegar. Do this daily for 30 days.

6) **Raw Egg Shampoo**

Ingredients:
- 1 organic pasture-raised raw egg
- Fresh squeezed juice of 1 organic lemon
- 2 tablespoons organic raw apple cider vinegar

<u>Instructions</u>:
Add egg, lemon juice, and apple cider vinegar into a 16oz glass mason jar. Seal, and shake very well. Take the shampoo into the shower, lather, and wash your hair.

Note: Make sure to rinse your hair only using cool water. If the water is too hot you'll end up cooking the egg, and later find pieces of egg in your hair.

7) <u>Raw Face Mask</u>
You can also apply this to your whole body, including cuts, wounds, and sunburn.

<u>Ingredients</u>:
- 3 tablespoons fresh organic grass-fed raw bone marrow
- 3 tablespoons organic grass-fed raw butter (softened)
- 3 tablespoons organic grass-fed raw cream
- 3 tablespoons fresh squeezed organic lemon juice

<u>Instructions</u>:
Allow marrow bone to soften by sitting on a counter for 30-60 minutes. Scrape the raw marrow from the inside of the bone. Add marrow, butter, cream, and lemon juice into a Vitamix blender and blend until it reaches a smooth consistency. Apply to your face. Relax, and remove the mask after 20 minutes. Place the remaining mask into an 8oz glass jar, and store in the refrigerator. Shelf life is 7 days.

8) <u>Cave Woman Cream</u>
This is a face and whole body cream. Even though it's not raw, it is still an excellent moisturizer.

Ingredients:
- 1 pint rendered organic grass-fed beef tallow
- 1/3 cup organic cold pressed olive oil
- 5ml organic Ylang Ylang essential oil (or your favorite scent)

Instructions:
Warm the tallow lightly on low heat in a pan until it becomes liquid. Do not allow to boil. Turn off the burner. Add olive oil and essential oil to the pan while stirring. Place in a glass jar. Shelf life is 6 months at room temperature.

Note: The tallow must be organic because conventional tallow may be full of chemicals, due to the fact that most toxins are stored in fat. You can purchase rendered beef tallow from a local butcher shop, or you can purchase suet (cow or sheep) and render it yourself.

9) Raw Ginger Butter Toothpaste

Ingredients:
- 2 tablespoons organic grass-fed raw butter (softened)
- ½ teaspoon organic ginger juice

Instructions:
Juice the ginger root in a home juicer, or grate it on a zester, and squeeze it through a metal tea strainer.

Place ginger juice into a 2oz glass jar, add butter, and mix well. Shelf life is 5 days at room temperature, or slightly longer in the refrigerator.

10) <u>Raw Toothpaste</u>

<u>Ingredients</u>:
- 1 tablespoon Bentonite Clay (must be a <u>fine</u> powder)
- 1 tablespoon organic turmeric powder
- 1 tablespoon organic raw coconut oil
- 5 drops organic peppermint essential oil

<u>Instructions</u>:
Add clay, turmeric powder, coconut oil, and peppermint oil into a glass bowl and mix together using a chopstick until it's smooth. Place mixture into a 4oz glass jar. Shelf life is 6 months at room temperature.

11) <u>Raw Honey Mask</u>

<u>Step 1</u>: **Steam Facial**
<u>Ingredients</u>:
- 2 cups filtered water

<u>Instructions</u>:
Add water to a medium sized pot, and bring to a boil. Turn the burner off, and place the pot on a counter. Put your face over the pot while allowing the steam to gently open the pores on your face. Continue for 5 minutes.

<u>Step 2</u>: **The Mask**
<u>Ingredients</u>:
- 1-2 tablespoons raw honey

Raw Paleo

<u>Instructions</u>:
Using your fingers, apply a thin coat of raw honey to your face. Relax for 15 minutes. Rinse the honey off with warm water.

References

(1) _Pottenger's cats: A Study in Nutrition_, Francis Pottenger, (1983)

(2) _The Real Truth about Vitamins and Antioxidants_, Judith De Cava (1997)

(3) _We Want to Live: The Primal Diet_, Aajonus Vonderplanitz, (1993)

(4) _Nutrition and Physical Degeneration_, Weston A. Price, DDS (1939)

(5) _Food is Your Best Medicine_, Henry Bieler, MD (1982)

(6) _Enzyme Nutrition_, Edward Howell, MD (1985)

(7) www.cholesterol-and-health.com, Chris Masterjon, PhD.

(8) _The Cholesterol Myths: Exposing the Fallacy That Saturated Fat and Cholesterol Cause Heart Disease_, Uffe Ravnskov, MD, PhD (2000)

(9) *The Great Cholesterol Con: The Truth About What Really Causes Heart Disease and How to Avoid It*, Malcolm Kendrick, MD (2007)

(10) www.anthonycolpo.com/new-study-women-with-higher-cholesterol-live-longer/, Anthony Colpo.

(11) *The curse of Louis Pasteur*. Appleton, N. (1999)

(12) *The Untold Story of Milk*, Ron Schmid, ND (2009)

(13) www.realmilk.com/health/milk-homogenization-and-heart-disease/ *Milk Homogenization and Heart Disease,* Mary Enig, PhD, (2013)

(14) *The Milk Book*, William Campbell Douglass, MD (1984)

(15) www.ncbi.nlm.nih.gov/pubmed/25550171, Curcumin boosts DHA in the brain: Implications for the prevention of anxiety disorders. 2015 May; 1852(5):951-61.

(16) *American Journal of Physical Medicine*, 1941, 133; Physiological Zoology, 1935 8:457.

(17) www.umaine.edu/publications/2258e/, Salmonella and Food Safety. Mahmoud El-Begearmi, (2011)

(18) https://foodpoisoningbulletin.com/2013/salmonella-is-naturally-occurring-in-animal-intestines/, Food Poisoning Bulletin, Salmonella is Naturally Occurring in Animal Intestines, Carla Gillepsie (2013)

(19) www.pbs.org/wgbh/pages/frontline/shows/meat/interviews/pollan.html, Modern Meat, Michael Pollan.

(20) www.doctor-natasha.com/, Natasha McBride, MD.

Made in the USA
Lexington, KY
15 May 2019